THE OFFICIAL PATIENT'S SOURCEBOOK

on

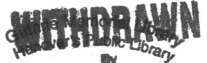
ADULT ACUTE LYMPHOBLASTIC LEUKEMIA

JAMES N. PARKER, M.D.
AND PHILIP M. PARKER, PH.D., EDITORS

ii

ICON Health Publications
ICON Group International, Inc.
7404 Trade Street
San Diego, CA 92121 USA

Last digit indicates print number: 10 9 8 7 6 4 5 3 2 1

Publisher, Health Care: Philip Parker, Ph.D.
Editor(s): James Parker, M.D., Philip Parker, Ph.D.

Publisher's note: The ideas, procedures, and suggestions contained in this book are not intended as a substitute for consultation with your physician. All matters regarding your health require medical supervision. As new medical or scientific information becomes available from academic and clinical research, recommended treatments and drug therapies may undergo changes. The authors, editors, and publisher have attempted to make the information in this book up to date and accurate in accord with accepted standards at the time of publication. The authors, editors, and publisher are not responsible for errors or omissions or for consequences from application of the book, and make no warranty, expressed or implied, in regard to the contents of this book. Any practice described in this book should be applied by the reader in accordance with professional standards of care used in regard to the unique circumstances that may apply in each situation, in close consultation with a qualified physician. The reader is advised to always check product information (package inserts) for changes and new information regarding dose and contraindications before taking any drug or pharmacological product. Caution is especially urged when using new or infrequently ordered drugs, herbal remedies, vitamins and supplements, alternative therapies, complementary therapies and medicines, and integrative medical treatments.

Cataloging-in-Publication Data

Parker, James N., 1961-
Parker, Philip M., 1960-

The Official Patient's Sourcebook on Adult Acute Lymphoblastic Leukemia: A Revised and Updated Directory for the Internet Age/James N. Parker and Philip M. Parker, editors
        p.   cm.
Includes bibliographical references, glossary and index.
ISBN: 0-497-11184-5
1. Adult Acute Lymphoblastic Leukemia-Popular works. I. Title.

Disclaimer

This publication is not intended to be used for the diagnosis or treatment of a health problem or as a substitute for consultation with licensed medical professionals. It is sold with the understanding that the publisher, editors, and authors are not engaging in the rendering of medical, psychological, financial, legal, or other professional services.

References to any entity, product, service, or source of information that may be contained in this publication should not be considered an endorsement, either direct or implied, by the publisher, editors or authors. ICON Group International, Inc., the editors, or the authors are not responsible for the content of any Web pages nor publications referenced in this publication.

Copyright Notice

Dedication

To the healthcare professionals dedicating their time and efforts to the study of adult acute lymphoblastic leukemia.

Acknowledgements

The collective knowledge generated from academic and applied research summarized in various references has been critical in the creation of this sourcebook which is best viewed as a comprehensive compilation and collection of information prepared by various official agencies which directly or indirectly are dedicated to adult acute lymphoblastic leukemia. All of the *Official Patient's Sourcebooks* draw from various agencies and institutions associated with the United States Department of Health and Human Services, and in particular, the Office of the Secretary of Health and Human Services (OS), the Administration for Children and Families (ACF), the Administration on Aging (AOA), the Agency for Healthcare Research and Quality (AHRQ), the Agency for Toxic Substances and Disease Registry (ATSDR), the Centers for Disease Control and Prevention (CDC), the Food and Drug Administration (FDA), the Healthcare Financing Administration (HCFA), the Health Resources and Services Administration (HRSA), the Indian Health Service (IHS), the institutions of the National Institutes of Health (NIH), the Program Support Center (PSC), and the Substance Abuse and Mental Health Services Administration (SAMHSA). In addition to these sources, information gathered from the National Library of Medicine, the United States Patent Office, the European Union, and their related organizations has been invaluable in the creation of this sourcebook. Some of the work represented was financially supported by the Research and Development Committee at INSEAD. This support is gratefully acknowledged. Finally, special thanks are owed to Tiffany Freeman for her excellent editorial support.

About the Editors

James N. Parker, M.D.

Dr. James N. Parker received his Bachelor of Science degree in Psychobiology from the University of California, Riverside and his M.D. from the University of California, San Diego. In addition to authoring numerous research publications, he has lectured at various academic institutions. Dr. Parker is the medical editor for the *Official Patient's Sourcebook* series published by ICON Health Publications.

Philip M. Parker, Ph.D.

Philip M. Parker is the Eli Lilly Chair Professor of Innovation, Business and Society at INSEAD (Fontainebleau, France and Singapore). Dr. Parker has also been Professor at the University of California, San Diego and has taught courses at Harvard University, the Hong Kong University of Science and Technology, the Massachusetts Institute of Technology, Stanford University, and UCLA. Dr. Parker is the associate editor for the *Official Patient's Sourcebook* series published by ICON Health Publications.

About ICON Health Publications

In addition to adult acute lymphoblastic leukemia, *Official Patient's Sourcebooks* are available for the following related topics:

- The Official Patient's Sourcebook on Adult Acute Myeloid Leukemia
- The Official Patient's Sourcebook on Adult Hodgkin's Disease
- The Official Patient's Sourcebook on Adult Non-Hodgkin's Lymphoma
- The Official Patient's Sourcebook on Chronic Lymphocytic Leukemia
- The Official Patient's Sourcebook on Chronic Myelogenous Leukemia
- The Official Patient's Sourcebook on Hairy Cell Leukemia
- The Official Patient's Sourcebook on Hodgkin's Disease during Pregnancy
- The Official Patient's Sourcebook on Multiple Myeloma and Other Plasma Cell Neoplasms
- The Official Patient's Sourcebook on Mycosis Fungoides and the Sezary Syndrome
- The Official Patient's Sourcebook on Myelodysplastic Syndromes
- The Official Patient's Sourcebook on Myeloproliferative Disorders
- The Official Patient's Sourcebook on Non-Hodgkin's Lymphoma during Pregnancy
- The Official Patient's Sourcebook on Primary CNS Lymphoma

To discover more about ICON Health Publications, simply check with your preferred online booksellers, including Barnes&Noble.com and Amazon.com which currently carry all of our titles. Or, feel free to contact us directly for bulk purchases or institutional discounts:

ICON Group International, Inc.
7404 Trade Street
San Diego, CA 92121 USA
Fax: 858-635-9414
Web site: **www.icongrouponline.com/health**

Table of Contents

INTRODUCTION

Overview

Dr. C. Everett Koop, former U.S. Surgeon General, once said, "The best prescription is knowledge."[1] The Agency for Healthcare Research and Quality (AHRQ) of the National Institutes of Health (NIH) echoes this view and recommends that every patient incorporate education into the treatment process. According to the AHRQ:

> Finding out more about your condition is a good place to start. By contacting groups that support your condition, visiting your local library, and searching on the Internet, you can find good information to help guide your treatment decisions. Some information may be hard to find—especially if you don't know where to look.[2]

As the AHRQ mentions, finding the right information is not an obvious task. Though many physicians and public officials had thought that the emergence of the Internet would do much to assist patients in obtaining reliable information, in March 2001 the National Institutes of Health issued the following warning:

> The number of Web sites offering health-related resources grows every day. Many sites provide valuable information, while others may have information that is unreliable or misleading.[3]

---

[1] Quotation from **http://www.drkoop.com**.
[2] The Agency for Healthcare Research and Quality (AHRQ):
http://www.ahcpr.gov/consumer/diaginfo.htm.
[3] From the NIH, National Cancer Institute (NCI):
http://cancertrials.nci.nih.gov/beyond/evaluating.html.

Since the late 1990s, physicians have seen a general increase in patient Internet usage rates. Patients frequently enter their doctor's offices with printed Web pages of home remedies in the guise of latest medical research. This scenario is so common that doctors often spend more time dispelling misleading information than guiding patients through sound therapies. *The Official Patient's Sourcebook on Adult Acute Lymphoblastic Leukemia* has been created for patients who have decided to make education and research an integral part of the treatment process. The pages that follow will tell you where and how to look for information covering virtually all topics related to adult acute lymphoblastic leukemia, from the essentials to the most advanced areas of research.

The title of this book includes the word "official." This reflects the fact that the sourcebook draws from public, academic, government, and peer-reviewed research. Selected readings from various agencies are reproduced to give you some of the latest official information available to date on adult acute lymphoblastic leukemia.

Given patients' increasing sophistication in using the Internet, abundant references to reliable Internet-based resources are provided throughout this sourcebook. Where possible, guidance is provided on how to obtain free-of-charge, primary research results as well as more detailed information via the Internet. E-book and electronic versions of this sourcebook are fully interactive with each of the Internet sites mentioned (clicking on a hyperlink automatically opens your browser to the site indicated). Hard copy users of this sourcebook can type cited Web addresses directly into their browsers to obtain access to the corresponding sites. Since we are working with ICON Health Publications, hard copy *Sourcebooks* are frequently updated and printed on demand to ensure that the information provided is current.

In addition to extensive references accessible via the Internet, every chapter presents a "Vocabulary Builder." Many health guides offer glossaries of technical or uncommon terms in an appendix. In editing this sourcebook, we have decided to place a smaller glossary within each chapter that covers terms used in that chapter. Given the technical nature of some chapters, you may need to revisit many sections. Building one's vocabulary of medical terms in such a gradual manner has been shown to improve the learning process.

We must emphasize that no sourcebook on adult acute lymphoblastic leukemia should affirm that a specific diagnostic procedure or treatment discussed in a research study, patent, or doctoral dissertation is "correct" or your best option. This sourcebook is no exception. Each patient is unique.

Deciding on appropriate options is always up to the patient in consultation with their physician and healthcare providers.

Organization

This sourcebook is organized into three parts. Part I explores basic techniques to researching adult acute lymphoblastic leukemia (e.g. finding guidelines on diagnosis, treatments, and prognosis), followed by a number of topics, including information on how to get in touch with organizations, associations, or other patient networks dedicated to adult acute lymphoblastic leukemia. It also gives you sources of information that can help you find a doctor in your local area specializing in treating adult acute lymphoblastic leukemia. Collectively, the material presented in Part I is a complete primer on basic research topics for patients with adult acute lymphoblastic leukemia.

Part II moves on to advanced research dedicated to adult acute lymphoblastic leukemia. Part II is intended for those willing to invest many hours of hard work and study. It is here that we direct you to the latest scientific and applied research on adult acute lymphoblastic leukemia. When possible, contact names, links via the Internet, and summaries are provided. It is in Part II where the vocabulary process becomes important as authors publishing advanced research frequently use highly specialized language. In general, every attempt is made to recommend "free-to-use" options.

Part III provides appendices of useful background reading for all patients with adult acute lymphoblastic leukemia or related disorders. The appendices are dedicated to more pragmatic issues faced by many patients with adult acute lymphoblastic leukemia. Accessing materials via medical libraries may be the only option for some readers, so a guide is provided for finding local medical libraries which are open to the public. Part III, therefore, focuses on advice that goes beyond the biological and scientific issues facing patients with adult acute lymphoblastic leukemia.

Scope

While this sourcebook covers adult acute lymphoblastic leukemia, your doctor, research publications, and specialists may refer to your condition using a variety of terms. Therefore, you should understand that adult acute lymphoblastic leukemia is often considered a synonym or a condition closely related to the following:

- Acute Lymphoblastic Leukemia
- Lymphoblastic Leukemia
- Lymphoid Leukemia

In addition to synonyms and related conditions, physicians may refer to adult acute lymphoblastic leukemia using certain coding systems. The International Classification of Diseases, 9th Revision, Clinical Modification (ICD-9-CM) is the most commonly used system of classification for the world's illnesses. Your physician may use this coding system as an administrative or tracking tool. The following classification is commonly used for adult acute lymphoblastic leukemia:[4]

- 204.0 acute lymphoblastic leukemia

For the purposes of this sourcebook, we have attempted to be as inclusive as possible, looking for official information for all of the synonyms relevant to adult acute lymphoblastic leukemia. You may find it useful to refer to synonyms when accessing databases or interacting with healthcare professionals and medical librarians.

Moving Forward

Since the 1980s, the world has seen a proliferation of healthcare guides covering most illnesses. Some are written by patients or their family members. These generally take a layperson's approach to understanding and coping with an illness or disorder. They can be uplifting, encouraging, and highly supportive. Other guides are authored by physicians or other healthcare providers who have a more clinical outlook. Each of these two styles of guide has its purpose and can be quite useful.

As editors, we have chosen a third route. We have chosen to expose you to as many sources of official and peer-reviewed information as practical, for the purpose of educating you about basic and advanced knowledge as recognized by medical science today. You can think of this sourcebook as your personal Internet age reference librarian.

---

[4] This list is based on the official version of the World Health Organization's 9th Revision, International Classification of Diseases (ICD-9). According to the National Technical Information Service, "ICD-9CM extensions, interpretations, modifications, addenda, or errata other than those approved by the U.S. Public Health Service and the Health Care Financing Administration are not to be considered official and should not be utilized. Continuous maintenance of the ICD-9-CM is the responsibility of the federal government."

Why "Internet age"? All too often, patients diagnosed with adult acute lymphoblastic leukemia will log on to the Internet, type words into a search engine, and receive several Web site listings which are mostly irrelevant or redundant. These patients are left to wonder where the relevant information is, and how to obtain it. Since only the smallest fraction of information dealing with adult acute lymphoblastic leukemia is even indexed in search engines, a non-systematic approach often leads to frustration and disappointment. With this sourcebook, we hope to direct you to the information you need that you would not likely find using popular Web directories. Beyond Web listings, in many cases we will reproduce brief summaries or abstracts of available reference materials. These abstracts often contain distilled information on topics of discussion.

While we focus on the more scientific aspects of adult acute lymphoblastic leukemia, there is, of course, the emotional side to consider. Later in the sourcebook, we provide a chapter dedicated to helping you find peer groups and associations that can provide additional support beyond research produced by medical science. We hope that the choices we have made give you the most options available in moving forward. In this way, we wish you the best in your efforts to incorporate this educational approach into your treatment plan.

The Editors

PART I: THE ESSENTIALS

ABOUT PART I

Part I has been edited to give you access to what we feel are "the essentials" on adult acute lymphoblastic leukemia. The essentials of a disease typically include the definition or description of the disease, a discussion of who it affects, the signs or symptoms associated with the disease, tests or diagnostic procedures that might be specific to the disease, and treatments for the disease. Your doctor or healthcare provider may have already explained the essentials of adult acute lymphoblastic leukemia to you or even given you a pamphlet or brochure describing adult acute lymphoblastic leukemia. Now you are searching for more in-depth information. As editors, we have decided, nevertheless, to include a discussion on where to find essential information that can complement what your doctor has already told you. In this section we recommend a process, not a particular Web site or reference book. The process ensures that, as you search the Web, you gain background information in such a way as to maximize your understanding.

CHAPTER 1. THE ESSENTIALS ON ADULT ACUTE LYMPHOBLASTIC LEUKEMIA: GUIDELINES

Overview

Official agencies, as well as federally funded institutions supported by national grants, frequently publish a variety of guidelines on adult acute lymphoblastic leukemia. These are typically called "Fact Sheets" or "Guidelines." They can take the form of a brochure, information kit, pamphlet, or flyer. Often they are only a few pages in length. The great advantage of guidelines over other sources is that they are often written with the patient in mind. Since new guidelines on adult acute lymphoblastic leukemia can appear at any moment and be published by a number of sources, the best approach to finding guidelines is to systematically scan the Internet-based services that post them.

The National Institutes of Health (NIH)[5]

The National Institutes of Health (NIH) is the first place to search for relatively current patient guidelines and fact sheets on adult acute lymphoblastic leukemia. Originally founded in 1887, the NIH is one of the world's foremost medical research centers and the federal focal point for medical research in the United States. At any given time, the NIH supports some 35,000 research grants at universities, medical schools, and other research and training institutions, both nationally and internationally. The rosters of those who have conducted research or who have received NIH support over the years include the world's most illustrious scientists and

---

[5] Adapted from the NIH: **http://www.nih.gov/about/NIHoverview.html**.

physicians. Among them are 97 scientists who have won the Nobel Prize for achievement in medicine.

There is no guarantee that any one Institute will have a guideline on a specific disease, though the National Institutes of Health collectively publish over 600 guidelines for both common and rare diseases. The best way to access NIH guidelines is via the Internet. Although the NIH is organized into many different Institutes and Offices, the following is a list of key Web sites where you are most likely to find NIH clinical guidelines and publications dealing with adult acute lymphoblastic leukemia and associated conditions:

- Office of the Director (OD); guidelines consolidated across agencies available at **http://www.nih.gov/health/consumer/conkey.htm**

- National Library of Medicine (NLM); extensive encyclopedia (A.D.A.M., Inc.) with guidelines available at **http://www.nlm.nih.gov/medlineplus/healthtopics.html**

- National Cancer Institute (NCI); guidelines available at **http://cancernet.nci.nih.gov/pdq/pdq_treatment.shtml**

Among the above, the National Cancer Institute (NCI) is particularly noteworthy. The NCI coordinates the National Cancer Program, which conducts and supports research, training, health information dissemination, and other programs with respect to the cause, diagnosis, prevention, and treatment of cancer, rehabilitation from cancer, and the continuing care of cancer patients and the families of cancer patients.[6] Specifically, the Institute:

- Supports and coordinates research projects conducted by universities, hospitals, research foundations, and businesses throughout this country and abroad through research grants and cooperative agreements.

- Conducts research in its own laboratories and clinics.

- Supports education and training in fundamental sciences and clinical disciplines for participation in basic and clinical research programs and treatment programs relating to cancer through career awards, training grants, and fellowships.

- Supports research projects in cancer control.

- Supports a national network of cancer centers.

- Collaborates with voluntary organizations and other national and foreign institutions engaged in cancer research and training activities.

---

[6] This paragraph has been adapted from the NCI: **http://www.nci.nih.gov/**. "Adapted" signifies that a passage has been reproduced exactly or slightly edited for this book.

- Encourages and coordinates cancer research by industrial concerns where such concerns evidence a particular capability for programmatic research.

- Collects and disseminates information on cancer.

- Supports construction of laboratories, clinics, and related facilities necessary for cancer research through the award of construction grants.

The following patient guideline was recently published by the NCI on adult acute lymphoblastic leukemia.

What Is Adult Acute Lymphoblastic Leukemia?[7]

Adult acute lymphoblastic leukemia (ALL) is a type of cancer in which the bone marrow makes too many lymphocytes (a type of white blood cell).

Adult acute lymphoblastic leukemia (ALL; also called acute lymphocytic leukemia) is a cancer of the blood and bone marrow. This type of cancer usually gets worse quickly if it is not treated.

Normally, the bone marrow produces stem cells (immature cells) that develop into mature blood cells. There are 3 types of mature blood cells:

- Red blood cells that carry oxygen and other materials to all tissues of the body.

- White blood cells that fight infection and disease.

- Platelets that help prevent bleeding by causing blood clots to form.

In ALL, too many stem cells develop into a type of white blood called lymphocytes. These lymphocytes may also be called lymphoblasts or leukemic cells.

There are 3 types of lymphocytes:

- B lymphocytes that make antibodies to help fight infection.

- T lymphocytes that help B lymphocytes make the antibodies that help fight infection.

- Natural killer cells that attack cells with cancer or a virus.

---

[7] The following guidelines appeared on the NCI Web site on February 9, 2004. The text was last modified in January 2004. The text has been adapted for this sourcebook.

- In ALL, the lymphocytes are not able to fight infection very well. Also, as the number of lymphocytes increases in the blood and bone marrow, there is less room for healthy white blood cells, red blood cells, and platelets. This may cause infection, anemia, and easy bleeding. The cancer can also spread to the central nervous system (brain and spinal cord).

Previous chemotherapy and exposure to radiation may affect the risk of developing ALL.

Possible risk factors for ALL include the following:

- Being male.
- Being white.
- Being older than 70 years of age.
- Past treatment with chemotherapy or radiation therapy.
- Exposure to atomic bomb radiation.
- Having a certain genetic disorder such as Down syndrome.

The early signs of ALL may be similar to the flu or other common diseases. A doctor should be consulted if any of the following problems occur:

- Weakness or feeling tired.
- Fever.
- Easy bruising or bleeding.
- Petechiae (flat, pinpoint spots under the skin caused by bleeding).
- Shortness of breath.
- Loss of appetite or weight loss.
- Pain in the bones or stomach.
- Pain or feeling of fullness below the ribs.
- Painless lumps in the neck, underarm, stomach, or groin.

These and other symptoms may be caused by adult acute lymphoblastic leukemia or by other conditions.

Tests that examine the blood and bone marrow are used to detect (find) and diagnose adult ALL.

The following tests and procedures may be used:

- Physical exam and history: An exam of the body to check general signs of health, including checking for signs of disease, such as lumps or anything else that seems unusual. A history of the patient's health habits and past illnesses and treatments will also be taken.

- Complete blood count: A procedure in which a sample of blood is drawn and checked for the following:

    - The number of red blood cells, white blood cells, and platelets.

    - The amount of hemoglobin (the protein that carries oxygen) in the red blood cells.

    - The portion of the blood sample made up of red blood cells.

- Peripheral blood smear: A procedure in which a sample of blood is checked for the presence of blast cells, number and kinds of white blood cells, the number of platelets, and changes in the shape of blood cells.

- Bone marrow biopsy and aspiration: The removal of a small piece of bone and bone marrow by inserting a needle into the hipbone or breastbone. A pathologist views the samples under a microscope to look for abnormal cells.

- Cytogenetic analysis: A test in which the cells in a sample of blood or bone marrow are looked at under a microscope to find out if there are certain changes in the chromosomes in the lymphocytes. For example, sometimes in ALL, part of one chromosome is moved to another chromosome. This is called the Philadelphia chromosome.

- Immunophenotyping: A test in which the cells in a sample of blood or bone marrow are looked at under a microscope to find out if malignant (cancerous) lymphocytes began from the B lymphocytes or the T lymphocytes.

Certain Factors Affecting Prognosis (Chance of Recovery) and Treatment Options

The prognosis (chance of recovery) and treatment options depend on the following:

- The age of the patient.

- Whether the cancer has spread to the brain or spinal cord.

- Whether the Philadelphia chromosome is present.

- Whether the cancer has been treated before or has recurred (come back).

Stages of Adult Acute Lymphoblastic Leukemia

Once adult ALL has been diagnosed, tests are done to find out if the cancer has spread to the central nervous system (brain and spinal cord) or to other parts of the body.

The extent or spread of cancer is usually described as stages. It is important to know whether the leukemia has spread outside the blood and bone marrow in order to plan treatment. The following tests and procedures may be used to determine if the leukemia has spread:

- Chest x-ray: An x-ray of the organs and bones inside the chest. An x-ray is a type of energy beam that can go through the body and onto film, making a picture of areas inside the body.

- Lumbar puncture: A procedure used to collect cerebrospinal fluid from the spinal column. This is done by placing a needle into the spinal column. This procedure is also called an LP or spinal tap.

- Ultrasound: A procedure in which high-energy sound waves (ultrasound) are bounced off internal tissues or organs in the abdomen and make echoes. The echoes form a picture of body tissues called a sonogram.

- CT scan (CAT scan): A procedure that makes a series of detailed pictures of the abdomen, taken from different angles. The pictures are made by a computer linked to an x-ray machine. A dye may be injected into a vein or swallowed to help the organs or tissues show up more clearly. This procedure is also called computed tomography, computerized tomography, or computerized axial tomography.

There is no standard staging system for adult ALL.

The disease is classified as untreated, in remission, or recurrent.

Untreated

- The ALL is newly diagnosed and has not been treated except to relieve symptoms such as fever, bleeding or pain.
- The complete blood count is abnormal.
- There are more than 5% blasts (leukemia cells) in the bone marrow.

- There are signs and symptoms of leukemia.

In Remission

- The ALL has been treated.
- The complete blood count is normal.
- There are less than 5% blasts (leukemia cells) in the bone marrow.
- There are no signs or symptoms of leukemia in the brain and spinal cord or elsewhere in the body.

Recurrent/Refractory

Recurrent disease means that the leukemia has come back after going into remission. Refractory disease means that the leukemia has failed to go into remission following treatment.

Treatment Option Overview

There are different types of treatment for patients with adult ALL.

Different types of treatment are available for patients with adult acute lymphoblastic leukemia (ALL). Some treatments are standard (the currently used treatment), and some are being tested in clinical trials. A treatment clinical trial is a research study meant to help improve current treatments or obtain information on new treatments for patients with cancer. When clinical trials show that a new treatment is better than the "standard" treatment, the new treatment may become the standard treatment.

Clinical trials are taking place in many parts of the country. Information about ongoing clinical trials is available from the NCI Cancer.gov Web site. Choosing the most appropriate cancer treatment is a decision that ideally involves the patient, family, and health care team.

The treatment of adult ALL usually has 2 phases.

The treatment of adult ALL is done in phases:

- Remission induction therapy: This is the first phase of treatment. Its purpose is to kill the leukemia cells in the blood and bone marrow. This puts the leukemia into remission.

- Maintenance therapy: This is the second phase of treatment. It begins once the leukemia is in remission. The purpose of maintenance therapy is to kill any remaining leukemia cells that may not be active but could begin to regrow and cause a relapse. This phase is also called remission continuation therapy.

Treatment called central nervous system (CNS) sanctuary therapy is usually given during each phase of therapy. Because chemotherapy that is given by mouth or injected into a vein may not reach leukemia cells in the CNS (brain and spinal cord), the cells are able to find "sanctuary" (hide) in the CNS. Intrathecal chemotherapy and radiation therapy are able to reach leukemia cells in the CNS and are given to kill the leukemia cells and prevent the cancer from recurring (coming back). CNS sanctuary therapy is also called CNS prophylaxis.

Three types of standard treatment are used:

Chemotherapy

Chemotherapy is a cancer treatment that uses drugs to stop the growth of cancer cells, either by killing the cells or by stopping the cells from dividing. When chemotherapy is taken by mouth or injected into a vein or muscle, the drugs enter the bloodstream and can reach cancer cells throughout the body (systemic chemotherapy). When chemotherapy is placed directly into the spinal column, a body cavity such as the abdomen, or an organ, the drugs mainly affect cancer cells in those areas. Combination chemotherapy is treatment using more than one anticancer drug. The way the chemotherapy is given depends on the type and stage of the cancer being treated.

Intrathecal chemotherapy may be used to treat adult ALL that has spread, or may spread, to the brain and spinal cord. When used to prevent cancer from spreading to the brain and spinal cord, it is called central nervous system (CNS) sanctuary therapy or CNS prophylaxis. Intrathecal chemotherapy is given in addition to chemotherapy by mouth or vein.

Radiation Therapy

Radiation therapy is a cancer treatment that uses high-energy x-rays or other types of radiation to kill cancer cells. There are two types of radiation therapy. External radiation therapy uses a machine outside the body to send radiation toward the cancer. Internal radiation therapy uses a radioactive substance sealed in needles, seeds, wires, or catheters that are placed directly into or near the cancer. External radiation therapy may be used to treat adult ALL that has spread, or may spread, to the brain and spinal cord. When used this way, it is called central nervous system (CNS) sanctuary therapy or CNS prophylaxis.

High-Dose Chemotherapy with Stem Cell Transplantation

Stem cell transplantation is a method of giving chemotherapy and replacing blood-forming cells destroyed by the cancer treatment. Stem cells (immature blood cells) are removed from the blood or bone marrow of a donor and are frozen for storage. After the chemotherapy is completed, the stored stem cells are thawed and given back to the patient through an infusion. These reinfused stem cells grow into (and restore) the body's blood cells.

Types of Treatment Being Tested in Clinical Trials

These include the following:

- Biologic therapy

Biologic therapy is a treatment that uses the patient's immune system to fight cancer. Substances made by the body or made in a laboratory are used to boost, direct, or restore the body's natural defenses against cancer. This type of cancer treatment is also called biotherapy or immunotherapy.

This summary section refers to specific treatments under study in clinical trials, but it may not mention every new treatment being studied. Information about ongoing clinical trials is available from the NCI Cancer.gov Web site.

Treatment by Stage

Treatment of adult ALL depends on the type of disease, the patient's age and overall condition.

Standard treatment may be considered based on its effectiveness in past studies, or participation in a clinical trial may be considered. Not all patients are cured with standard therapy, and some standard treatments may have more side effects than are desired. For these reasons, clinical trials are designed to find better ways to treat cancer patients and are based on the most up-to-date information. Clinical trials are ongoing in most parts of the country for most stages of ALL. For more information, call the Cancer Information Service at 1-800-4-CANCER (1-800-422-6237); TTY at 1-800-332-8615.

Untreated Adult Acute Lymphoblastic Leukemia

Standard treatment of adult acute lymphoblastic leukemia (ALL) during the remission induction phase includes the following:

- Combination chemotherapy.
- CNS prophylaxis therapy including chemotherapy (intrathecal and/or systemic) with or without radiation therapy to the brain.

Adult Acute Lymphoblastic Leukemia in Remission

Standard treatment of adult ALL during the maintenance phase includes the following:

- Combination chemotherapy.
- High-dose chemotherapy with stem cell transplantation.
- CNS prophylaxis therapy including chemotherapy (intrathecal and/or systemic) with or without radiation therapy to the brain.

Recurrent Adult Acute Lymphoblastic Leukemia

Standard treatment of recurrent adult ALL may include the following:

- Combination chemotherapy followed by stem cell transplantation.
- Low-dose radiation therapy as palliative care to relieve symptoms and improve the quality of life.

Some of the treatments being studied in clinical trials for recurrent adult ALL include the following:

- A clinical trial of stem cell transplantation using the patient's own stem cells.
- A clinical trial of biologic therapy.
- A clinical trial of new chemotherapy drugs.

To Learn More

Call

For more information, U.S. residents may call the National Cancer Institute's (NCI's) Cancer Information Service toll-free at 1-800-4-CANCER (1-800-422-6237), Monday through Friday from 9:00 a.m. to 4:30 p.m. Deaf and hard-of-hearing callers with TTY equipment may call 1-800-332-8615. The call is free and a trained Cancer Information Specialist is available to answer your questions.

Web Sites and Organizations

The NCI's Cancer.gov Web site (**http://cancer.gov**) provides online access to information on cancer, clinical trials, and other Web sites and organizations that offer support and resources for cancer patients and their families. There are also many other places where people can get materials and information about cancer treatment and services. Local hospitals may have information on local and regional agencies that offer information about finances, getting to and from treatment, receiving care at home, and dealing with problems associated with cancer treatment.

Publications

The NCI has booklets and other materials for patients, health professionals, and the public. These publications discuss types of cancer, methods of cancer treatment, coping with cancer, and clinical trials. Some publications provide information on tests for cancer, cancer causes and prevention, cancer statistics, and NCI research activities. NCI materials on these and other topics may be ordered online or printed directly from the NCI Publications Locator (**https://cissecure.nci.nih.gov/ncipubs**). These materials can also be ordered by telephone from the Cancer Information Service toll-free at 1-800-4-CANCER (1-800-422-6237), TTY at 1-800-332-8615.

LiveHelp

The NCI's LiveHelp service, a program available on several of the Institute's Web sites, provides Internet users with the ability to chat online with an Information Specialist. The service is available from Monday - Friday 9:00

AM - 10:00 PM Eastern Time. Information Specialists can help Internet users find information on NCI Web sites and answer questions about cancer.

Write

For more information from the NCI, please write to this address:

National Cancer Institute
Office of Communications
31 Center Drive, MSC 2580
Bethesda, MD 20892-2580

About PDQ

PDQ Is a Comprehensive Cancer Database Available on Cancer.gov

PDQ is the National Cancer Institute's (NCI's) comprehensive cancer information database. Most of the information contained in PDQ is available online at Cancer.gov (**http://cancer.gov**), the NCI's Web site. PDQ is provided as a service of the NCI. The NCI is part of the National Institutes of Health, the federal government's focal point for biomedical research.

PDQ Contains Cancer Information Summaries

The PDQ database contains summaries of the latest published information on cancer prevention, detection, genetics, treatment, supportive care, and complementary and alternative medicine. Most summaries are available in two versions. The health professional versions provide detailed information written in technical language. The patient versions are written in easy-to-understand, non-technical language. Both versions provide current and accurate cancer information.

The PDQ cancer information summaries are developed by cancer experts and reviewed regularly. Editorial Boards made up of experts in oncology and related specialties are responsible for writing and maintaining the cancer information summaries. The summaries are reviewed regularly and changes are made as new information becomes available. The date on each summary ("Date Last Modified") indicates the time of the most recent change.

PDQ Contains Information on Clinical Trials

Before starting treatment, patients may want to think about taking part in a clinical trial. A clinical trial is a study to answer a scientific question, such as whether one treatment is better than another. Trials are based on past studies and what has been learned in the laboratory. Each trial answers certain scientific questions in order to find new and better ways to help cancer patients. During treatment clinical trials, information is collected about new treatments, the risks involved, and how well they do or do not work. If a clinical trial shows that a new treatment is better than one currently being used, the new treatment may become "standard."

Listings of clinical trials are included in PDQ and are available online at Cancer.gov (**http://cancer.gov/clinical_trials**). Descriptions of the trials are available in health professional and patient versions. Many cancer doctors who take part in clinical trials are also listed in PDQ. For more information, call the Cancer Information Service at 1-800-4-CANCER (1-800-422-6237); TTY at 1-800-332-8615.

More Guideline Sources

The guideline above on adult acute lymphoblastic leukemia is only one example of the kind of material that you can find online and free of charge. The remainder of this chapter will direct you to other sources which either publish or can help you find additional guidelines on topics related to adult acute lymphoblastic leukemia. Many of the guidelines listed below address topics that may be of particular relevance to your specific situation or of special interest to only some patients with adult acute lymphoblastic leukemia. Due to space limitations these sources are listed in a concise manner. Do not hesitate to consult the following sources by either using the Internet hyperlink provided, or, in cases where the contact information is provided, contacting the publisher or author directly.

Topic Pages: MEDLINEplus

For patients wishing to go beyond guidelines published by specific Institutes of the NIH, the National Library of Medicine has created a vast and patient-oriented healthcare information portal called MEDLINEplus. Within this Internet-based system are "health topic pages." You can think of a health topic page as a guide to patient guides. To access this system, log on to **http://www.nlm.nih.gov/medlineplus/healthtopics.html**. From there you can either search using the alphabetical index or browse by broad topic areas. Recently, MEDLINEplus listed the following as being relevant to adult acute lymphoblastic leukemia:

Bone Marrow Diseases
http://www.nlm.nih.gov/medlineplus/bonemarrowdiseases.html

Lymphoma
http://www.nlm.nih.gov/medlineplus/lymphoma.html

You may also choose to use the search utility provided by MEDLINEplus at the following Web address: **http://www.nlm.nih.gov/medlineplus/**. Simply type a keyword into the search box and click "Search." This utility is similar to the NIH search utility, with the exception that it only includes materials that are linked within the MEDLINEplus system (mostly patient-oriented information). It also has the disadvantage of generating unstructured results. We recommend, therefore, that you use this method only if you have a very targeted search.

The NIH Search Utility

After browsing the references listed at the beginning of this chapter, you may want to explore the NIH search utility. This allows you to search for documents on over 100 selected Web sites that comprise the NIH-WEB-SPACE. Each of these servers is "crawled" and indexed on an ongoing basis. Your search will produce a list of various documents, all of which will relate in some way to adult acute lymphoblastic leukemia. The drawbacks of this approach are that the information is not organized by theme and that the references are often a mix of information for professionals and patients. Nevertheless, a large number of the listed Web sites provide useful background information. We can only recommend this route, therefore, for relatively rare or specific disorders, or when using highly targeted searches. To use the NIH search utility, visit the following Web page: **http://search.nih.gov/index.html**.

Additional Web Sources

A number of Web sites that often link to government sites are available to the public. These can also point you in the direction of essential information. The following is a representative sample:

- AOL: **http://search.aol.com/cat.adp?id=168&layer=&from=subcats**

- Family Village: **http://www.familyvillage.wisc.edu/specific.htm**

- Google: **http://directory.google.com/Top/Health/Conditions_and_Diseases/**

- Med Help International: **http://www.medhelp.org/HealthTopics/A.html**

- Open Directory Project: **http://dmoz.org/Health/Conditions_and_Diseases/**

- Yahoo.com: **http://dir.yahoo.com/Health/Diseases_and_Conditions/**

- WebMD®Health: **http://my.webmd.com/health_topics**

Vocabulary Builder

The material in this chapter may have contained a number of unfamiliar words. The following Vocabulary Builder introduces you to terms used in this chapter that have not been covered in the previous chapter:

Catheters: A small, flexible tube that may be inserted into various parts of the body to inject or remove liquids. [NIH]

Genetics: The biological science that deals with the phenomena and mechanisms of heredity. [NIH]

Lymphoblastic: One of the most aggressive types of non-Hodgkin lymphoma. [NIH]

Lymphoblasts: Interferon produced predominantly by leucocyte cells. [NIH]

Lymphoma: Tumor of lymphatic tissue. [NIH]

Specialist: In medicine, one who concentrates on 1 special branch of medical science. [NIH]

CHAPTER 2. SEEKING GUIDANCE

Overview

Some patients are comforted by the knowledge that a number of organizations dedicate their resources to helping people with adult acute lymphoblastic leukemia. These associations can become invaluable sources of information and advice. Many associations offer aftercare support, financial assistance, and other important services. Furthermore, healthcare research has shown that support groups often help people to better cope with their conditions.[8] In addition to support groups, your physician can be a valuable source of guidance and support. Therefore, finding a physician that can work with your unique situation is a very important aspect of your care.

In this chapter, we direct you to resources that can help you find patient organizations and medical specialists. We begin by describing how to find associations and peer groups that can help you better understand and cope with adult acute lymphoblastic leukemia. The chapter ends with a discussion on how to find a doctor that is right for you.

Finding Associations

There are a several Internet directories that provide lists of medical associations with information on or resources relating to adult acute lymphoblastic leukemia. By consulting all of associations listed in this chapter, you will have nearly exhausted all sources for patient associations concerned with adult acute lymphoblastic leukemia.

---

[8] Churches, synagogues, and other houses of worship might also have groups that can offer you the social support you need.

The National Cancer Institute (NCI)

The National Cancer Institute (NCI) has complied a list of national organizations that offer services to people with cancer and their families. To view the list, see the NCI fact sheet online at the following Web address: **http://cis.nci.nih.gov/fact/8_1.htm**. The name of each organization is accompanied by its contact information and a brief explanation of its services.

The National Health Information Center (NHIC)

The National Health Information Center (NHIC) offers a free referral service to help people find organizations that provide information about adult acute lymphoblastic leukemia. For more information, see the NHIC's Web site at **http://www.health.gov/NHIC/** or contact an information specialist by calling 1-800-336-4797.

DIRLINE

A comprehensive source of information on associations is the DIRLINE database maintained by the National Library of Medicine. The database comprises some 10,000 records of organizations, research centers, and government institutes and associations which primarily focus on health and biomedicine. DIRLINE is available via the Internet at the following Web site: **http://dirline.nlm.nih.gov/**. Simply type in "adult acute lymphoblastic leukemia" (or a synonym) or the name of a topic, and the site will list information contained in the database on all relevant organizations.

The Combined Health Information Database

Another comprehensive source of information on healthcare associations is the Combined Health Information Database. Using the "Detailed Search" option, you will need to limit your search to "Organizations" and "adult acute lymphoblastic leukemia". Type the following hyperlink into your Web browser: **http://chid.nih.gov/detail/detail.html**. To find associations, use the drop boxes at the bottom of the search page where "You may refine your search by." For publication date, select "All Years." Then, select your preferred language and the format option "Organization Resource Sheet." By making these selections and typing in "adult acute lymphoblastic leukemia" (or synonyms) into the "For these words:" box, you will only receive results on organizations dealing with adult acute lymphoblastic leukemia. You should check back periodically with this database since it is updated every 3 months.

The National Organization for Rare Disorders, Inc.

The National Organization for Rare Disorders, Inc. has prepared a Web site that provides, at no charge, lists of associations organized by specific diseases. You can access this database at the following Web site: **http://www.rarediseases.org/search/orgsearch.html**. Type "adult acute lymphoblastic leukemia" (or a synonym) in the search box, and click "Submit Query."

Cancer Support Groups[9]

People diagnosed with cancer and their families face many challenges that may leave them feeling overwhelmed, afraid, and alone. It can be difficult to cope with these challenges or to talk to even the most supportive family members and friends. Often, support groups can help people affected by cancer feel less alone and can improve their ability to deal with the uncertainties and challenges that cancer brings. Support groups give people who are affected by similar diseases an opportunity to meet and discuss ways to cope with the illness.

How Can Support Groups Help?

People who have been diagnosed with cancer sometimes find they need assistance coping with the emotional as well as the practical aspects of their disease. In fact, attention to the emotional burden of cancer is sometimes part of a patient's treatment plan. Cancer support groups are designed to provide a confidential atmosphere where cancer patients or cancer survivors can discuss the challenges that accompany the illness with others who may have experienced the same challenges. For example, people gather to discuss the emotional needs created by cancer, to exchange information about their disease — including practical problems such as managing side effects or returning to work after treatment — and to share their feelings. Support

---

[9] This section has been adapted from the NCI: **http://cis.nci.nih.gov/fact/8_8.htm**.

groups have helped thousands of people cope with these and similar situations.

Can Family Members and Friends Participate in Support Groups?

Family and friends are affected when cancer touches someone they love, and they may need help in dealing with stresses such as family disruptions, financial worries, and changing roles within relationships. To help meet these needs, some support groups are designed just for family members of people diagnosed with cancer; other groups encourage families and friends to participate along with the cancer patient or cancer survivor.

How Can People Find Support Groups?

Many organizations offer support groups for people diagnosed with cancer and their family members or friends. The NCI fact sheet *National Organizations That Offer Services to People with Cancer and Their Families* lists many cancer-concerned organizations that can provide information about support groups. This fact sheet is available at **http://cis.nci.nih.gov/fact/8_1.htm** on the Internet, or can be ordered from the Cancer Information Service at 1–800–4–CANCER (1–800–422–6237). Some of these organizations provide information on their Web sites about contacting support groups.

Doctors, nurses, or hospital social workers who work with cancer patients may also have information about support groups, such as their location, size, type, and how often they meet. Most hospitals have social services departments that provide information about cancer support programs. Additionally, many newspapers carry a special health supplement containing information about where to find support groups.

What Types of Support Groups Are Available?

Several kinds of support groups are available to meet the individual needs of people at all stages of cancer treatment, from diagnosis through follow-up care. Some groups are general cancer support groups, while more specialized groups may be for teens or young adults, for family members, or for people affected by a particular disease. Support groups may be led by a professional, such as a psychiatrist, psychologist, or social worker, or by cancer patients or survivors. In addition, support groups can vary in approach, size, and how often they meet. Many groups are free, but some require a fee (people can contact their health insurance company to find out whether their plan will cover the cost). It is important for people to find an atmosphere that is comfortable and meets their individual needs.

Online Support Groups

In addition to support groups, commercial Internet service providers offer forums and chat rooms for people with different illnesses and conditions. WebMD®, for example, offers such a service at their Web site: **http://boards.webmd.com/roundtable**. These online self-help communities can help you connect with a network of people whose concerns are similar to yours. Online support groups are places where people can talk informally. If you read about a novel approach, consult with your doctor or other healthcare providers, as the treatments or discoveries you hear about may not be scientifically proven to be safe and effective.

The Cancer Information Service[10]

The Cancer Information Service (CIS) is a program of the National Cancer Institute (NCI), the Nation's lead agency for cancer research. As a resource for information and education about cancer, the CIS is a leader in helping people become active participants in their own health care by providing the latest information on cancer in understandable language. Through its network of regional offices, the CIS serves the United States, Puerto Rico, the U.S. Virgin Islands, and the Pacific Islands.

For 25 years, the Cancer Information Service has provided the latest and most accurate cancer information to patients and families, the public, and health professionals by:

- Interacting with people one-on-one through its Information Service,

- Working with organizations through its Partnership Program,

- Participating in research efforts to find the best ways to help people adopt healthier behaviors,

- Providing access to NCI information over the Internet.

---

[10] This section has been adapted from the NCI: **http://cis.nci.nih.gov/fact/2_5.htm**.

How Does the CIS Assist the Public?

Through the CIS toll-free telephone service (1–800–4–CANCER), callers speak with knowledgeable, caring staff who are experienced at explaining medical information in easy-to-understand terms. CIS information specialists answer calls in English and Spanish. They also provide cancer information to deaf and hard of hearing callers through the toll-free TTY number (1–800–332–8615). CIS staff have access to comprehensive, accurate information from the NCI on a range of cancer topics, including the most recent advances in cancer treatment. They take as much time as each caller needs, provide thorough and personalized attention, and keep all calls confidential.

The CIS also provides live, online assistance to users of NCI Web sites through LiveHelp, an instant messaging service that is available from 9:00 a.m. to 7:30 p.m. Eastern time, Monday through Friday. Through LiveHelp, information specialists provide answers to questions about cancer and help in navigating Cancer.gov, the NCI's Web site.

Through the telephone numbers or LiveHelp service, CIS users receive:

- Answers to their questions about cancer, including ways to prevent cancer, symptoms and risks, diagnosis, current treatments, and research studies;

- Written materials from the NCI;

- Referrals to clinical trials and cancer-related services, such as treatment centers, mammography facilities, or other cancer organizations;

- Assistance in quitting smoking from information specialists trained in smoking cessation counseling.

What Kind of Assistance Does the CIS Partnership Program Offer?

Through its Partnership Program, the CIS collaborates with established national, state, and regional organizations to reach minority and medically underserved audiences with cancer information. Partnership Program staff provide assistance to organizations developing programs that focus on breast and cervical cancer, clinical trials, tobacco control, and cancer awareness for special populations. To reach those in need, the CIS:

- Helps bring cancer information to people who do not traditionally seek health information or who may have difficulties doing so because of educational, financial, cultural, or language barriers;

- Provides expertise to organizations to help strengthen their ability to inform people they serve about cancer; and

- Links organizations with similar goals and helps them plan and evaluate programs, develop coalitions, conduct training on cancer-related topics, and use NCI resources.

How Do CIS Research Efforts Assist the Public?

The CIS plays an important role in research by studying the most effective ways to communicate with people about healthy lifestyles; health risks; and options for preventing, diagnosing, and treating cancer. The ability to conduct health communications research is a unique aspect of the CIS. Results from these research studies can be applied to improving the way the CIS communicates about cancer and can help other programs communicate more effectively.

How Do People Reach the Cancer Information Service?

- To speak with a CIS information specialist call 1–800–4–CANCER (1–800–422–6237), 9:00 a.m. to 4:30 p.m. local time, Monday through Friday. Deaf or hard of hearing callers with TTY equipment may call 1–800–332–8615.

- To obtain online assistance visit the NCI's Cancer Information Web site at **http://cancer.gov/cancer_information** and click on the LiveHelp link between 9:00 a.m. and 7:30 p.m. Eastern time, Monday through Friday.

- For information 24 hours a day, 7 days a week call 1–800–4–CANCER and select option 4 to hear recorded information at any time.

- Visit NCI's Web site at **http://cancer.gov** on the Internet.

- Visit the CIS Web site at **http://cancer.gov/cis** on the Internet.

Finding Cancer Resources in Your Community[11]

If you have cancer or are undergoing cancer treatment, there are places in your community to turn to for help. There are many local organizations throughout the country that offer a variety of practical and support services to people with cancer. However, people often don't know about these services or are unable to find them. National cancer organizations can assist

---

[11] Adapted from the NCI: **http://cis.nci.nih.gov/fact/8_9.htm**.

you in finding these resources, and there are a number of things you can do for yourself.

Whether you are looking for a support group, counseling, advice, financial assistance, transportation to and from treatment, or information about cancer, most neighborhood organizations, local health care providers, or area hospitals are a good place to start. Often, the hardest part of looking for help is knowing the right questions to ask.

What Kind of Help Can I Get?

Until now, you probably never thought about the many issues and difficulties that arise with a diagnosis of cancer. There are support services to help you deal with almost any type of problem that might occur. The first step in finding the help you need is knowing what types of services are available. The following pages describe some of these services and how to find them.

- **Information on Cancer.** Most national cancer organizations provide a range of information services, including materials on different types of cancer, treatments, and treatment-related issues.

- **Counseling.** While some people are reluctant to seek counseling, studies show that having someone to talk to reduces stress and helps people both mentally and physically. Counseling can also provide emotional support to cancer patients and help them better understand their illness. Different types of counseling include individual, group, family, self-help (sometimes called peer counseling), bereavement, patient-to-patient, and sexuality.

- **Medical Treatment Decisions.** Often, people with cancer need to make complicated medical decisions. Many organizations provide hospital and physician referrals for second opinions and information on clinical trials (research studies with people), which may expand treatment options.

- **Prevention and Early Detection.** While cancer prevention may never be 100 percent effective, many things (such as quitting smoking and eating healthy foods) can greatly reduce a person's risk for developing cancer. Prevention services usually focus on smoking cessation and nutrition. Early detection services, which are designed to detect cancer when a person has no symptoms of disease, can include referrals for screening mammograms, Pap tests, or prostate exams.

- **Home Health Care.** Home health care assists patients who no longer need to stay in a hospital or nursing home, but still require professional medical help. Skilled nursing care, physical therapy, social work services, and nutrition counseling are all available at home.

- **Hospice Care.** Hospice is care focused on the special needs of terminally ill cancer patients. Sometimes called *palliative care*, it centers around providing comfort, controlling physical symptoms, and giving emotional support to patients who can no longer benefit from curative treatment. Hospice programs provide services in various settings, including the patient's home, hospice centers, hospitals, or skilled nursing facilities. Your doctor or social worker can provide a referral for these services.

- **Rehabilitation.** Rehabilitation services help people adjust to the effects of cancer and its treatment. Physical rehabilitation focuses on recovery from the physical effects of surgery or the side effects associated with chemotherapy. Occupational or vocational therapy helps people readjust to everyday routines, get back to work, or find employment.

- **Advocacy.** Advocacy is a general term that refers to promoting or protecting the rights and interests of a certain group, such as cancer patients. Advocacy groups may offer services to assist with legal, ethical, medical, employment, legislative, or insurance issues, among others. For instance, if you feel your insurance company has not handled your claim fairly, you may want to advocate for a review of its decision.

- **Financial.** Having cancer can be a tremendous financial burden to cancer patients and their families. There are programs sponsored by the government and nonprofit organizations to help cancer patients with problems related to medical billing, insurance coverage, and reimbursement issues. There are also sources for financial assistance, and ways to get help collecting entitlements from Medicaid, Medicare, and the Social Security Administration.

- **Housing/Lodging.** Some organizations provide lodging for the family of a patient undergoing treatment, especially if it is a child who is ill and the parents are required to accompany the child to treatment.

- **Children's Services.** A number of organizations provide services for children with cancer, including summer camps, make-a-wish programs, and help for parents seeking child care.

How to Find These Services

Often, the services that people with cancer are looking for are right in their own neighborhood or city. The following is a list of places where you can begin your search for help.

- The hospital, clinic, or medical center where you see your doctor, received your diagnosis, or where you undergo treatment should be able to give you information. Your doctor or nurse may be able to tell you about your specific medical condition, pain management, rehabilitation services, home nursing, or hospice care.

- Most hospitals also have a social work, home care, or discharge planning department. This department may be able to help you find a support group, a nonprofit agency that helps people who have cancer, or the government agencies that oversee Social Security, Medicare, and Medicaid. While you are undergoing treatment, be sure to ask the hospital about transportation, practical assistance, or even temporary child care. Talk to a hospital financial counselor in the business office about developing a monthly payment plan if you need help with hospital expenses.

- The public library is an excellent source of information, as are patient libraries at many cancer centers. A librarian can help you find books and articles through a literature search.

- A local church, synagogue, YMCA or YWCA, or fraternal order may provide financial assistance, or may have volunteers who can help with transportation and home care. Catholic Charities, the United Way, or the American Red Cross may also operate local offices. Some of these organizations may provide home care, and the United Way's information and referral service can refer you to an agency that provides financial help. To find the United Way serving your community, visit their online directory at **http://www.unitedway.org** on the Internet or look in the White Pages of your local telephone book.

- Local or county government agencies may offer low-cost transportation (sometimes called para-transit) to individuals unable to use public transportation. Most states also have an Area Agency on Aging that offers low-cost services to people over 60. Your hospital or community social worker can direct you to government agencies for entitlements, including Social Security, state disability, Medicaid, income maintenance, and food stamps. (Keep in mind that most applications to entitlement programs take some time to process.) The Federal government also runs the Hill-Burton program (1–800–638–0742), which funds certain medical facilities and hospitals to provide cancer patients with free or low-cost care if they are in financial need.

Getting the Most From a Service: What To Ask

No matter what type of help you are looking for, the only way to find resources to fit your needs is to ask the right questions. When you are calling an organization for information, it is important to think about what questions you are going to ask before you call. Many people find it helpful to write out their questions in advance, and to take notes during the call. Another good tip is to ask the name of the person with whom you are speaking in case you have follow-up questions. Below are some of the questions you may want to consider if you are calling or visiting a new agency and want to learn about how they can help:

- How do I apply [for this service]?

- Are there eligibility requirements? What are they?

- Is there an application process? How long will it take? What information will I need to complete the application process? Will I need anything else to get the service?

- Do you have any other suggestions or ideas about where I can find help?

The most important thing to remember is that you will rarely receive help unless you ask for it. In fact, asking can be the hardest part of getting help. Don't be afraid or ashamed to ask for assistance. Cancer is a very difficult disease, but there are people and services that can ease your burdens and help you focus on your treatment and recovery.

Finding Doctors Who Specialize in Cancer Care[12]

One of the most important aspects of your treatment will be the relationship between you and your doctor or specialist. All patients with adult acute lymphoblastic leukemia must go through the process of selecting a physician. A common way to find a doctor who specializes in cancer care is to ask for a referral from your primary care physician. Sometimes, you may know a specialist yourself, or through the experience of a family member, coworker, or friend.

The following resources may also be able to provide you with names of doctors who specialize in treating specific diseases or conditions. However, these resources may not have information about the quality of care that the doctors provide.

---

[12] Adapted from the NCI: **http://cis.nci.nih.gov/fact/7_47.htm**.

- Your local hospital or its patient referral service may be able to provide you with a list of specialists who practice at that hospital.

- Your nearest National Cancer Institute (NCI)-designated cancer center can provide information about doctors who practice at that center. The NCI fact sheet *The National Cancer Institute Cancer Centers Program* describes and gives contact information, including Web sites, for NCI-designated cancer treatment centers around the country. Many of the cancer centers' Web sites have searchable directories of physicians who practice at each facility. The NCI's fact sheet is available at **http://cis.nci.nih.gov/fact/1_2.htm** on the Internet, or by calling the Cancer Information Service (CIS) at 1–800–4–CANCER (1–800–422–6237).

- The American Board of Medical Specialties (ABMS) publishes a list of board-certified physicians. The *Official ABMS Directory of Board Certified Medical Specialists* lists doctors' names along with their specialty and their educational background. This resource is available in most public libraries. The ABMS also has a Web site that can be used to verify whether a specific physician is board-certified. This free service is located at **http://www.abms.org/newsearch.asp** on the Internet. Verification of a physician's board certification can also be obtained by calling the ABMS at 1–866–275–2267 (1–866–ASK–ABMS).

- The American Medical Association (AMA) provides an online service called AMA Physician Select that offers basic professional information on virtually every licensed physician in the United States and its possessions. The database can be searched by doctor's name or by medical specialty. The AMA Physician Select service is located at **http://www.ama-assn.org/aps/amahg.htm** on the Internet.

- The American Society of Clinical Oncologists (ASCO) provides an online list of doctors who are members of ASCO. The member database has the names and affiliations of over 15,000 oncologists worldwide. It can be searched by doctor's name, institution's name, location, and/or type of board certification. This service is located at **http://www.asco.org/people/db/html/m_db.htm** on the Internet.

- The American College of Surgeons (ACOS) Fellowship Database is an online list of surgeons who are Fellows of the ACOS. The list can be searched by doctor's name, geographic location, or medical specialty. This service is located at **http://web.facs.org/acsdir/default.htm** on the Internet. The ACOS can be contacted at 633 North Saint Clair Street, Chicago, IL 60611–3211; or by telephone at 312–202–5000.

- Local medical societies may maintain lists of doctors in each specialty.

- Public and medical libraries may have print directories of doctors' names, listed geographically by specialty.

- Your local Yellow Pages may have doctors listed by specialty under "Physicians."

The Agency for Healthcare Research and Quality (AHRQ) offers *Your Guide to Choosing Quality Health Care*, which has information for consumers on choosing a health plan, a doctor, a hospital, or a long-term care provider. The Guide includes suggestions and checklists that you can use to determine which doctor or hospital is best for you. This resource is available at **http://www.ahrq.gov/consumer/qntool.htm** on the Internet. You can also order the Guide by calling the AHRQ Publications Clearinghouse at 1–800–358–9295.

If you are a member of a health insurance plan, your choice may be limited to doctors who participate in your plan. Your insurance company can provide you with a list of participating primary care doctors and specialists. It is important to ask your insurance company if the doctor you choose is accepting new patients through your health plan. You also have the option of seeing a doctor outside your health plan and paying the costs yourself. If you have a choice of health insurance plans, you may first wish to consider which doctor or doctors you would like to use, then choose a plan that includes your chosen physician(s).

The National Comprehensive Cancer Network (NCCN) Physician Directory lists specialists who practice in the NCCN's 19 member institutions across the U.S. To access the directory, go to **http://www.nccn.org/** and click on "Physician Directory". To use this service, you will be required to scroll to the bottom of the page and select "I agree." Enter your search criteria and select "Find" at the bottom of the page. To obtain more information on a physician or institution, contact the institution's Physician Referral Department or the NCCN Patient Information and Referral Service at 1-888-909-NCCN or **patientinformation@nccn.org**.

If the previous sources did not meet your needs, you may want to log on to the Web site of the National Organization for Rare Disorders (NORD) at **http://www.rarediseases.org/**. NORD maintains a database of doctors with expertise in various rare diseases. The Metabolic Information Network (MIN), 800-945-2188, also maintains a database of physicians with expertise in various metabolic diseases.

Selecting Your Doctor[13]

When you have compiled a list of prospective doctors, call each of their offices. First, ask if the doctor accepts your health insurance plan and if he or she is taking new patients. If the doctor is not covered by your plan, ask yourself if you are prepared to pay the extra costs. The next step is to schedule a visit with your chosen physician. During the first visit you will have the opportunity to evaluate your doctor and to find out if you feel comfortable with him or her. Ask yourself, did the doctor:

- Give me a chance to ask questions about adult acute lymphoblastic leukemia?

- Really listen to my questions?

- Answer in terms I understood?

- Show respect for me?

- Ask me questions?

- Make me feel comfortable?

- Address the health problem(s) I came with?

- Ask me my preferences about different kinds of treatments for adult acute lymphoblastic leukemia?

- Spend enough time with me?

Trust your instincts when deciding if the doctor is right for you. But remember, it might take time for the relationship to develop. It takes more than one visit for you and your doctor to get to know each other.

Working with Your Doctor[14]

Research has shown that patients who have good relationships with their doctors tend to be more satisfied with their care and have better results. Here are some tips to help you and your doctor become partners:

- You know important things about your symptoms and your health history. Tell your doctor what you think he or she needs to know.

---

[13] This section has been adapted from the AHRQ: **www.ahrq.gov/consumer/qntascii/qntdr.htm.**
[14] This section has been adapted from the AHRQ: **www.ahrq.gov/consumer/qntascii/qntdr.htm.**

- It is important to tell your doctor personal information, even if it makes you feel embarrassed or uncomfortable.

- Bring a "health history" list with you (and keep it up to date).

- Always bring any medications you are currently taking with you to the appointment, or you can bring a list of your medications including dosage and frequency information. Talk about any allergies or reactions you have had to your medications.

- Tell your doctor about any natural or alternative medicines you are taking.

- Bring other medical information, such as x-ray films, test results, and medical records.

- Ask questions. If you don't, your doctor will assume that you understood everything that was said.

- Write down your questions before your visit. List the most important ones first to make sure that they are addressed.

- Consider bringing a friend with you to the appointment to help you ask questions. This person can also help you understand and/or remember the answers.

- Ask your doctor to draw pictures if you think that this would help you understand.

- Take notes. Some doctors do not mind if you bring a tape recorder to help you remember things, but always ask first.

- Let your doctor know if you need more time. If there is not time that day, perhaps you can speak to a nurse or physician assistant on staff or schedule a telephone appointment.

- Take information home. Ask for written instructions. Your doctor may also have brochures and audio and videotapes that can help you.

- After leaving the doctor's office, take responsibility for your care. If you have questions, call. If your symptoms get worse or if you have problems with your medication, call. If you had tests and do not hear from your doctor, call for your test results. If your doctor recommended that you have certain tests, schedule an appointment to get them done. If your doctor said you should see an additional specialist, make an appointment.

By following these steps, you will enhance the relationship you will have with your physician.

Finding a Cancer Treatment Facility[15]

Choosing a treatment facility is another important consideration for getting the best medical care possible. Although you may not be able to choose which hospital treats you in an emergency, you can choose a facility for scheduled and ongoing care. If you have already found a doctor for your cancer treatment, you may need to choose a facility based on where your doctor practices. Your doctor may be able to recommend a facility that provides quality care to meet your needs. You may wish to ask the following questions when considering a treatment facility:

- Has the facility had experience and success in treating my condition?

- Has the facility been rated by state, consumer, or other groups for its quality of care?

- How does the facility check and work to improve its quality of care?

- Has the facility been approved by a nationally recognized accrediting body, such as the American College of Surgeons (ACOS) and/or the Joint Commission on Accredited Healthcare Organizations (JCAHO)?

- Does the facility explain patients' rights and responsibilities? Are copies of this information available to patients?

- Does the treatment facility offer support services, such as social workers and resources to help me find financial assistance if I need it?

- Is the facility conveniently located?

If you are a member of a health insurance plan, your choice of treatment facilities may be limited to those that participate in your plan. Your insurance company can provide you with a list of approved facilities. Although the costs of cancer treatment can be very high, you have the option of paying out-of-pocket if you want to use a treatment facility that is not covered by your insurance plan. If you are considering paying for treatment yourself, you may wish to discuss the potential costs with your doctor beforehand. You may also want to speak with the person who does the billing for the treatment facility. In some instances, nurses and social workers can provide you with more information about coverage, eligibility, and insurance issues.

The following resources may help you find a hospital or treatment facility for your care:

---

[15] Adapted from the NCI: **http://cis.nci.nih.gov/fact/7_47.htm**. At this Web site, information on how to find treatment facilities is also available for patients living outside the U.S.

- The NCI fact sheet *The National Cancer Institute Cancer Centers Program* describes and gives contact information for NCI-designated cancer treatment centers around the country.

- The ACOS accredits cancer programs at hospitals and other treatment facilities. More than 1,400 programs in the United States have been designated by the ACOS as Approved Cancer Programs. The ACOS Web site offers a searchable database of these programs at **http://web.facs.org/cpm/default.htm** on the Internet. The ACOS can be contacted at 633 North Saint Clair Street, Chicago, IL 60611-3211; or by telephone at 312-202-5000.

- The JCAHO is an independent, not-for-profit organization that evaluates and accredits health care organizations and programs in the United States. It also offers information for the general public about choosing a treatment facility. The JCAHO Web site is located at **http://www.jcaho.org** on the Internet. The JCAHO is located at One Renaissance Boulevard, Oakbrook Terrace, IL 60181-4294. The telephone number is 630-792-5800.

- The JCAHO offers an online Quality Check service that patients can use to determine whether a specific facility has been accredited by the JCAHO and view the organization's performance reports. This service is located at **http://www.jcaho.org/qualitycheck/directry/directry.asp** on the Internet.

- The AHRQ publication *Your Guide To Choosing Quality Health Care* has suggestions and checklists for choosing the treatment facility that is right for you.

Additional Cancer Support Information

In addition to the references above, the NCI has set up guidance Web sites that offers information on issues relating to cancer. These include:

- Facing Forward - A Guide for Cancer Survivors:
  http://www.cancer.gov/cancer_information/doc_img.aspx?viewid=cc93a843-6fc0-409e-8798-5c65afc172fe

- Taking Time: Support for People With Cancer and the People Who Care About Them:
  http://www.cancer.gov/cancer_information/doc_img.aspx?viewid=21a46445-a5c8-4fee-95a3-d9d0d665077a

- When Cancer Recurs: Meeting the Challenge:
  **http://www.cancer.gov/cancer_information/doc_img.aspx?viewid=9e13
  d0d2-b7de-4bd6-87da-5750300a0dab**

- Your Health Care Team: Your Doctor Is Only the Beginning:
  http://cis.nci.nih.gov/fact/8_10.htm

Vocabulary Builder

The following vocabulary builder provides definitions of words used in this chapter that have not been defined in previous chapters:

Consultation: A deliberation between two or more physicians concerning the diagnosis and the proper method of treatment in a case. [NIH]

Hospice: Institution dedicated to caring for the terminally ill. [NIH]

PART II: ADDITIONAL RESOURCES AND ADVANCED MATERIAL

ABOUT PART II

In Part II, we introduce you to additional resources and advanced research on adult acute lymphoblastic leukemia. All too often, patients who conduct their own research are overwhelmed by the difficulty in finding and organizing information. The purpose of the following chapters is to provide you an organized and structured format to help you find additional information resources on adult acute lymphoblastic leukemia. In Part II, as in Part I, our objective is not to interpret the latest advances on adult acute lymphoblastic leukemia or render an opinion. Rather, our goal is to give you access to original research and to increase your awareness of sources you may not have already considered. In this way, you will come across the advanced materials often referred to in pamphlets, books, or other general works. Once again, some of this material is technical in nature, so consultation with a professional familiar with adult acute lymphoblastic leukemia is suggested.

CHAPTER 3. STUDIES ON ADULT ACUTE LYMPHOBLASTIC LEUKEMIA

Overview

Every year, academic studies are published on adult acute lymphoblastic leukemia or related conditions. Broadly speaking, there are two types of studies. The first are peer reviewed. Generally, the content of these studies has been reviewed by scientists or physicians. Peer-reviewed studies are typically published in scientific journals and are usually available at medical libraries. The second type of studies is non-peer reviewed. These works include summary articles that do not use or report scientific results. These often appear in the popular press, newsletters, or similar periodicals.

In this chapter, we will show you how to locate peer-reviewed references and studies on adult acute lymphoblastic leukemia. We will begin by discussing research that has been summarized and is free to view by the public via the Internet. We then show you how to generate a bibliography on adult acute lymphoblastic leukemia and teach you how to keep current on new studies as they are published or undertaken by the scientific community.

Federally Funded Research on Adult Acute Lymphoblastic Leukemia

The U.S. Government supports a variety of research studies relating to adult acute lymphoblastic leukemia and associated conditions. These studies are tracked by the Office of Extramural Research at the National Institutes of

Health.[16] CRISP (Computerized Retrieval of Information on Scientific Projects) is a searchable database of federally funded biomedical research projects conducted at universities, hospitals, and other institutions. Visit CRISP at **http://crisp.cit.nih.gov/crisp/crisp_query.generate_screen**. You can perform targeted searches by various criteria including geography, date, as well as topics related to adult acute lymphoblastic leukemia and related conditions.

For most of the studies, the agencies reporting into CRISP provide summaries or abstracts. As opposed to clinical trial research using patients, many federally funded studies use animals or simulated models to explore adult acute lymphoblastic leukemia and related conditions. In some cases, therefore, it may be difficult to understand how some basic or fundamental research could eventually translate into medical practice.

E-Journals: PubMed Central[17]

PubMed Central (PMC) is a digital archive of life sciences journal literature developed and managed by the National Center for Biotechnology Information (NCBI) at the U.S. National Library of Medicine (NLM).[18] Access to this growing archive of e-journals is free and unrestricted.[19] To search, go to **http://www.ncbi.nlm.nih.gov/entrez/query.fcgi?db=Pmc**, and type "adult acute lymphoblastic leukemia" (or synonyms) into the search box. This search gives you access to full-text articles. The following is a sample of items found for adult acute lymphoblastic leukemia in the PubMed Central database:

---

[16] Healthcare projects are funded by the National Institutes of Health (NIH), Substance Abuse and Mental Health Services (SAMHSA), Health Resources and Services Administration (HRSA), Food and Drug Administration (FDA), Centers for Disease Control and Prevention (CDCP), Agency for Healthcare Research and Quality (AHRQ), and Office of Assistant Secretary of Health (OASH).

[17] Adapted from the National Library of Medicine: **http://www.pubmedcentral.nih.gov/about/intro.html**.

[18] With PubMed Central, NCBI is taking the lead in preservation and maintenance of open access to electronic literature, just as NLM has done for decades with printed biomedical literature. PubMed Central aims to become a world-class library of the digital age.

[19] The value of PubMed Central, in addition to its role as an archive, lies the availability of data from diverse sources stored in a common format in a single repository. Many journals already have online publishing operations, and there is a growing tendency to publish material online only, to the exclusion of print.

- **AF5q31, a newly identified AF4-related gene, is fused to MLL in infant acute lymphoblastic leukemia with ins(5;11)(q31;q13q23).** by Taki T, Kano H, Taniwaki M, Sako M, Yanagisawa M, Hayashi Y.; 1999 Dec 7; http://www.pubmedcentral.gov/articlerender.fcgi?tool=pmcentrez&artid=24471

- **Characterization of the immunoglobulin heavy chain complementarity determining region (CDR)-III sequences from human B cell precursor acute lymphoblastic leukemia cells.** by Kiyoi H, Naoe T, Horibe K, Ohno R.; 1992 Mar; http://www.pubmedcentral.gov/picrender.fcgi?tool=pmcentrez&blobtype

- **Clonal analysis of childhood acute lymphoblastic leukemia with "cytogenetically independent" cell populations.** by Pui CH, Raskind WH, Kitchingman GR, Raimondi SC, Behm FG, Murphy SB, Crist WM, Fialkow PJ, Williams DL.; 1989 Jun; http://www.pubmedcentral.gov/picrender.fcgi?tool=pmcentrez&blobtype

- **Common acute lymphoblastic leukemia antigen (CALLA) is active neutral endopeptidase 24.11 ("enkephalinase"): direct evidence by cDNA transfection analysis.** by Shipp MA, Vijayaraghavan J, Schmidt EV, Masteller EL, D'Adamio L, Hersh LB, Reinherz EL.; 1989 Jan; http://www.pubmedcentral.gov/picrender.fcgi?tool=pmcentrez&blobtype

- **Common acute lymphoblastic leukemia antigen expressed on leukemia and melanoma cell lines has neutral endopeptidase activity.** by Jongeneel CV, Quackenbush EJ, Ronco P, Verroust P, Carrel S, Letarte M.; 1989 Feb; http://www.pubmedcentral.gov/picrender.fcgi?tool=pmcentrez&blobtype

- **DNA-binding and transcriptional regulatory properties of hepatic leukemia factor (HLF) and the t(17;19) acute lymphoblastic leukemia chimera E2A-HLF.** by Hunger SP, Brown R, Cleary ML.; 1994 Sep; http://www.pubmedcentral.gov/picrender.fcgi?tool=pmcentrez&blobtype

- **Folate pathway gene expression differs in subtypes of acute lymphoblastic leukemia and influences methotrexate pharmacodynamics.** by Kager L, Cheok M, Yang W, Zaza G, Cheng Q, Panetta JC, Pui CH, Downing JR, Relling MV, Evans WE.; 2005 Jan 3; http://www.pubmedcentral.gov/articlerender.fcgi?tool=pmcentrez&artid=539195

- **Growth Suppression of Pre-T Acute Lymphoblastic Leukemia Cells by Inhibition of Notch Signaling.** by Weng AP, Nam Y, Wolfe MS, Pear WS, Griffin JD, Blacklow SC, Aster JC.; 2003 Jan; http://www.pubmedcentral.gov/articlerender.fcgi?tool=pmcentrez&arti d=151540

- **Identification of two related markers for common acute lymphoblastic leukemia as heat shock proteins.** by Strahler JR, Kuick R, Eckerskorn C, Lottspeich F, Richardson BC, Fox DA, Stoolman LM, Hanson CA, Nichols D, Tueche HJ.; 1990 Jan; http://www.pubmedcentral.gov/picrender.fcgi?tool=pmcentrez&blobty pe

- **Impaired expression of interleukin 2 receptor and CD45RO antigen on lymphocytes from children with acute lymphoblastic leukemia in response to cytomegalovirus and varicella-zoster virus.** by Mizutani K, Ito M, Nakano T, Kamiya H, Sakurai M.; 1995 May; http://www.pubmedcentral.gov/articlerender.fcgi?tool=pmcentrez&ren dertype

- **Near-precise interchromosomal recombination and functional DNA topoisomerase II cleavage sites at MLL and AF-4 genomic breakpoints in treatment-related acute lymphoblastic leukemia with t(4;11) translocation.** by Lovett BD, Lo Nigro L, Rappaport EF, Blair IA, Osheroff N, Zheng N, Megonigal MD, Williams WR, Nowell PC, Felix CA.; 2001 Aug 14; http://www.pubmedcentral.gov/articlerender.fcgi?tool=pmcentrez&arti d=55533

- **Organization of the gene encoding common acute lymphoblastic leukemia antigen (neutral endopeptidase 24.11): multiple miniexons and separate 5' untranslated regions.** by D'Adamio L, Shipp MA, Masteller EL, Reinherz EL.; 1989 Sep; http://www.pubmedcentral.gov/picrender.fcgi?tool=pmcentrez&blobty pe

- **P53 mutation in acute T cell lymphoblastic leukemia is of somatic origin and is stable during establishment of T cell acute lymphoblastic leukemia cell lines.** by Yeargin J, Cheng J, Yu AL, Gjerset R, Bogart M, Haas M.; 1993 May; http://www.pubmedcentral.gov/picrender.fcgi?tool=pmcentrez&blobty pe

- **Polymorphisms of methylenetetrahydrofolate reductase (MTHFR) and susceptibility to pediatric acute lymphoblastic leukemia in a German study population.** by Schnakenberg E, Mehles A, Cario G, Rehe K,

Seidemann K, Schlegelberger B, Elsner HA, Welte KH, Schrappe M, Stanulla M.; 2005;
http://www.pubmedcentral.gov/articlerender.fcgi?tool=pmcentrez&arti
d=1164414

- **Stroma-supported culture in childhood B-lineage acute lymphoblastic leukemia cells predicts treatment outcome.** by Kumagai M, Manabe A, Pui CH, Behm FG, Raimondi SC, Hancock ML, Mahmoud H, Crist WM, Campana D.; 1996 Feb 1;
  http://www.pubmedcentral.gov/articlerender.fcgi?tool=pmcentrez&ren
  dertype

- **TAL1 and LIM-Only Proteins Synergistically Induce Retinaldehyde Dehydrogenase 2 Expression in T-Cell Acute Lymphoblastic Leukemia by Acting as Cofactors for GATA3.** by Ono Y, Fukuhara N, Yoshie O.; 1998 Dec;
  http://www.pubmedcentral.gov/articlerender.fcgi?tool=pmcentrez&arti
  d=109277

- **Tal-1 induces T cell acute lymphoblastic leukemia accelerated by casein kinase IIalpha.** by Kelliher MA, Seldin DC, Leder P.; 1996 Oct 1;
  http://www.pubmedcentral.gov/picrender.fcgi?tool=pmcentrez&blobty
  pe

- **The t(10;14)(q24;q11) of T-cell acute lymphoblastic leukemia juxtaposes the delta T-cell receptor with TCL3, a conserved and activated locus at 10q24.** by Zutter M, Hockett RD, Roberts CW, McGuire EA, Bloomstone J, Morton CC, Deaven LL, Crist WM, Carroll AJ, Korsmeyer SJ.; 1990 Apr;
  http://www.pubmedcentral.gov/picrender.fcgi?tool=pmcentrez&blobty
  pe

- **The t(11;14)(p15;q11) in a T-cell acute lymphoblastic leukemia cell line activates multiple transcripts, including Ttg-1, a gene encoding a potential zinc finger protein.** by McGuire EA, Hockett RD, Pollock KM, Bartholdi MF, O'Brien SJ, Korsmeyer SJ.; 1989 May;
  http://www.pubmedcentral.gov/picrender.fcgi?tool=pmcentrez&blobty
  pe

- **The t(14;21)(q11.2;q22) chromosomal translocation associated with T-cell acute lymphoblastic leukemia activates the BHLHB1 gene.** by Wang J, Jani-Sait SN, Escalon EA, Carroll AJ, de Jong PJ, Kirsch IR, Aplan PD.; 2000 Mar 28;
  http://www.pubmedcentral.gov/articlerender.fcgi?tool=pmcentrez&arti
  d=16268

The National Library of Medicine: PubMed

One of the quickest and most comprehensive ways to find academic studies in both English and other languages is to use PubMed, maintained by the National Library of Medicine. The advantage of PubMed over previously mentioned sources is that it covers a greater number of domestic and foreign references. It is also free to the public.[20] If the publisher has a Web site that offers full text of its journals, PubMed will provide links to that site, as well as to sites offering other related data. User registration, a subscription fee, or some other type of fee may be required to access the full text of articles in some journals.

To generate your own bibliography of studies dealing with adult acute lymphoblastic leukemia, simply go to the PubMed Web site at **www.ncbi.nlm.nih.gov/pubmed**. Type "adult acute lymphoblastic leukemia" (or synonyms) into the search box, and click "Go." The following is the type of output you can expect from PubMed for "adult acute lymphoblastic leukemia" (hyperlinks lead to article summaries):

- **A case of monosomy 20 in an adult acute lymphoblastic leukemia.Cancer Genet Cytogenet.**
  Author(s): Bonet C, Sole F, Woessner S, Florensa L, Besses C, Sans-Sabrafen J.
  Source: Cancer Genetics and Cytogenetics.
  http://www.ncbi.nlm.nih.gov/entrez/query.fcgi?cmd=Retrieve&db=pubmed&dopt=Abstract&list_uids=8402561&query_hl=1

- **A complex karyotype involving chromosomes 3, 6, 11, 12, and 22 in adult acute lymphoblastic leukemia.Leuk Lymphoma.**
  Author(s): Shivakumara S, Mathew S, Dalton J, Chandy M, Srivastava A.
  Source: Leukemia & Lymphoma.
  http://www.ncbi.nlm.nih.gov/entrez/query.fcgi?cmd=Retrieve&db=pubmed&dopt=Abstract&list_uids=12400611&query_hl=1

---

[20] PubMed was developed by the National Center for Biotechnology Information (NCBI) at the National Library of Medicine (NLM) at the National Institutes of Health (NIH). The PubMed database was developed in conjunction with publishers of biomedical literature as a search tool for accessing literature citations and linking to full-text journal articles at Web sites of participating publishers. Publishers that participate in PubMed supply NLM with their citations electronically prior to or at the time of publication.

- **A comprehensive genetic classification of adult acute lymphoblastic leukemia (ALL): analysis of the GIMEMA 0496 protocol.Blood.**
  Author(s): Mancini M, Scappaticci D, Cimino G, Nanni M, Derme V, Elia L, Tafuri A, Vignetti M, Vitale A, Cuneo A, Castoldi G, Saglio G, Pane F, Mecucci C, Camera A, Specchia G, Tedeschi A, Di Raimondo F, Fioritoni G, Fabbiano F, Marmont F, Ferrara F, Cascavilla N, Todeschini G, Nobile F, Kropp MG, Leoni P, Tabilio A, Luppi M, Annino L, Mandelli F, Foa R.
  Source: Blood.
  http://www.ncbi.nlm.nih.gov/entrez/query.fcgi?cmd=Retrieve&db=pubmed&dopt=Abstract&list_uids=15650057&query_hl=1

- **A phase II "window" study of topotecan in untreated patients with high risk adult acute lymphoblastic leukemia.Clin Cancer Res.**
  Author(s): Gore SD, Rowinsky EK, Miller CB, Griffin C, Chen TL, Borowitz M, Donehower RC, Burks KL, Armstrong DK, Burke PJ, Grever MR, Kaufmann SH.
  Source: Clinical Cancer Research : an Official Journal of the American Association for Cancer Research.
  http://www.ncbi.nlm.nih.gov/entrez/query.fcgi?cmd=Retrieve&db=pubmed&dopt=Abstract&list_uids=9829730&query_hl=1

- **A phase II study of high dose ARA-C and mitoxantrone for treatment of relapsed or refractory adult acute lymphoblastic leukemia.Leuk Res.**
  Author(s): Rosen PJ, Rankin C, Head DR, Boldt DH, Luthardt FW, Norwood T, Pugh RP, Karanes C, Appelbaum FR.
  Source: Leukemia Research.
  http://www.ncbi.nlm.nih.gov/entrez/query.fcgi?cmd=Retrieve&db=pubmed&dopt=Abstract&list_uids=10738999&query_hl=1

- **A randomized trial of induction therapy (daunorubicin, vincristine, prednisone versus daunorubicin, vincristine, prednisone, cytarabine and 6-thioguanine) in adult acute lymphoblastic leukemia with long-term follow-up: an Eastern Cooperative Oncology Group Study (E3486).Leuk Lymphoma.**
  Author(s): Wiernik PH, Cassileth PA, Leong T, Hoagland HC, Bennett JM, Paietta E, Oken MM; Eastern Cooperative Oncology Group Study.
  Source: Leukemia & Lymphoma.
  http://www.ncbi.nlm.nih.gov/entrez/query.fcgi?cmd=Retrieve&db=pubmed&dopt=Abstract&list_uids=14565653&query_hl=1

- **A report from the LALA-94 and LALA-SA groups on hypodiploidy with 30 to 39 chromosomes and near-triploidy: 2 possible expressions of a sole entity conferring poor prognosis in adult acute lymphoblastic leukemia (ALL).Blood.**
  Author(s): Charrin C, Thomas X, Ffrench M, Le QH, Andrieux J, Mozziconacci MJ, Lai JL, Bilhou-Nabera C, Michaux L, Bernheim A, Bastard C, Mossafa H, Perot C, Maarek O, Boucheix C, Lheritier V, Delannoy A, Fiere D, Dastugue N.
  Source: Blood.
  http://www.ncbi.nlm.nih.gov/entrez/query.fcgi?cmd=Retrieve&db=pubmed&dopt=Abstract&list_uids=15039281&query_hl=1

- **Addition of etoposide to initial therapy of adult acute lymphoblastic leukemia: a combined clinical and laboratory study.Leuk Lymphoma.**
  Author(s): Kaufmann SH, Karp JE, Burke PJ, Gore SD.
  Source: Leukemia & Lymphoma.
  http://www.ncbi.nlm.nih.gov/entrez/query.fcgi?cmd=Retrieve&db=pubmed&dopt=Abstract&list_uids=9021688&query_hl=1

- **Adolescent and adult acute lymphoblastic leukemia: prognostic features and outcome of therapy. A study of 293 patients.Blood.**
  Author(s): Baccarani M, Corbelli G, Amadori S, Drenthe-Schonk A, Willemze R, Meloni G, Cardozo PL, Haanen C, Mandelli F, Tura S.
  Source: Blood.
  http://www.ncbi.nlm.nih.gov/entrez/query.fcgi?cmd=Retrieve&db=pubmed&dopt=Abstract&list_uids=6954995&query_hl=1

- **Adriamycin in combination chemotherapy of adult acute lymphoblastic leukemia: a Southwest Oncology Group study.Med Pediatr Oncol.**
  Author(s): Shaw MT, Raab SO.
  Source: Medical and Pediatric Oncology.
  http://www.ncbi.nlm.nih.gov/entrez/query.fcgi?cmd=Retrieve&db=pubmed&dopt=Abstract&list_uids=284167&query_hl=1

- **Adult acute lymphoblastic leukemia at relapse. Cytogenetic, immunophenotypic, and molecular changes.Cancer.**
  Author(s): Chucrallah AE, Stass SA, Huh YO, Albitar M, Kantarjian HM.
  Source: Cancer.
  http://www.ncbi.nlm.nih.gov/entrez/query.fcgi?cmd=Retrieve&db=pubmed&dopt=Abstract&list_uids=8625224&query_hl=1

- **Adult acute lymphoblastic leukemia phenotypes defined by monoclonal antibodies.Blood.**
  Author(s): Sobol RE, Royston I, LeBien TW, Minowada J, Anderson K, Davey FR, Cuttner J, Schiffer C, Ellison RR, Bloomfield CD.
  Source: Blood.
  http://www.ncbi.nlm.nih.gov/entrez/query.fcgi?cmd=Retrieve&db=pubmed&dopt=Abstract&list_uids=3855666&query_hl=1

- **Adult acute lymphoblastic leukemia. Response to therapy according to presenting features in 62 patients.Eur J Cancer Clin Oncol.**
  Author(s): Lazzarino M, Morra E, Alessandrino EP, Canevari A, Salvaneschi L, Castelli G, Brusamolino E, Pagnucco G, Isernia P, Orlandi E, Zei G, Bernasconi C.
  Source: European Journal of Cancer & Clinical Oncology.
  http://www.ncbi.nlm.nih.gov/entrez/query.fcgi?cmd=Retrieve&db=pubmed&dopt=Abstract&list_uids=6961037&query_hl=1

- **Adult acute lymphoblastic leukemia.J Pak Med Assoc.**
  Author(s): Adil SN, Usman M.
  Source: Jpma. the Journal of the Pakistan Medical Association.
  http://www.ncbi.nlm.nih.gov/entrez/query.fcgi?cmd=Retrieve&db=pubmed&dopt=Abstract&list_uids=15518363&query_hl=1

- **Adult acute lymphoblastic leukemia: a multicentric randomized trial testing bone marrow transplantation as postremission therapy. The French Group on Therapy for Adult Acute Lymphoblastic Leukemia.J Clin Oncol.**
  Author(s): Fiere D, Lepage E, Sebban C, Boucheix C, Gisselbrecht C, Vernant JP, Varet B, Broustet A, Cahn JY, Rigal-Huguet F, et al.
  Source: Journal of Clinical Oncology : Official Journal of the American Society of Clinical Oncology.
  http://www.ncbi.nlm.nih.gov/entrez/query.fcgi?cmd=Retrieve&db=pubmed&dopt=Abstract&list_uids=8410124&query_hl=1

- **Adult acute lymphoblastic leukemia: description and analysis of long-term survivors. A retrospective study.Haematologica.**
  Author(s): Giona F, Mazzucconi MG, Aloe Spiriti MA, Defazio D, De Luca AM, Ferrazza G, Martinelli E, Mandelli F.
  Source: Haematologica.
  http://www.ncbi.nlm.nih.gov/entrez/query.fcgi?cmd=Retrieve&db=pubmed&dopt=Abstract&list_uids=2511117&query_hl=1

- **Adult acute lymphoblastic leukemia: results of an aggressive regimen in India.Leuk Lymphoma.**
  Author(s): Raje N, Pai S, Vaidya S, Gopal R, Parikh P, Saikia T, Pai V, Nadkarni K, Advani IM.
  Source: Leukemia & Lymphoma.
  http://www.ncbi.nlm.nih.gov/entrez/query.fcgi?cmd=Retrieve&db=pu
  bmed&dopt=Abstract&list_uids=7950917&query_hl=1

- **Adult acute lymphoblastic leukemia: results of the Iowa HOP-L protocol.J Clin Oncol.**
  Author(s): Radford JE Jr, Burns CP, Jones MP, Gingrich RD, Kemp JD, Edwards RW, McFadden DB, Dick FR, Wen BC.
  Source: Journal of Clinical Oncology : Official Journal of the American Society of Clinical Oncology.
  http://www.ncbi.nlm.nih.gov/entrez/query.fcgi?cmd=Retrieve&db=pu
  bmed&dopt=Abstract&list_uids=2642541&query_hl=1

- **Adult acute lymphoblastic leukemia--lineage specific classification of 30 cases.Taiwan Yi Xue Hui Za Zhi.**
  Author(s): Cheng AL, Chen YC, Wang CH, Shen MC, Hsieh RP, Tien HF, Liu MC, Lai HS, Liu CH.
  Source: Taiwan Yi Xue Hui Za Zhi. Journal of the Formosan Medical Association.
  http://www.ncbi.nlm.nih.gov/entrez/query.fcgi?cmd=Retrieve&db=pu
  bmed&dopt=Abstract&list_uids=2950202&query_hl=1

- **Age-adapted induction treatment of acute lymphoblastic leukemia in the elderly and assessment of maintenance with interferon combined with chemotherapy. A multicentric prospective study in forty patients. French Group for Treatment of Adult Acute Lymphoblastic Leukemia.Leukemia.**
  Author(s): Delannoy A, Sebban C, Cony-Makhoul P, Cazin B, Cordonnier C, Bouabdallah R, Cahn JY, Dreyfus F, Sadoun A, Vernant JP, Gay C, Broustet A, Michaux JL, Fiere D.
  Source: Leukemia : Official Journal of the Leukemia Society of America, Leukemia Research Fund, U.K.
  http://www.ncbi.nlm.nih.gov/entrez/query.fcgi?cmd=Retrieve&db=pu
  bmed&dopt=Abstract&list_uids=9305593&query_hl=1

- **Aggressive treatment improves survival in adult acute lymphoblastic leukemia.Eur J Haematol.**
  Author(s): Smedmyr B, Killander A, Simonsson B, Sundstrom C.
  Source: European Journal of Haematology.
  http://www.ncbi.nlm.nih.gov/entrez/query.fcgi?cmd=Retrieve&db=pu bmed&dopt=Abstract&list_uids=3208869&query_hl=1

- **Allogeneic bone marrow transplantation for adult acute lymphoblastic leukemia in first complete remission: factors predictive of transplant-related mortality and influence of total body irradiation modalities.Bone Marrow Transplant.**
  Author(s): Sutton L, Kuentz M, Cordonnier C, Blaise D, Devergie A, Guyotat D, Leblond V, Flesch M, Bordigoni P, Attal M, et al.
  Source: Bone Marrow Transplantation.
  http://www.ncbi.nlm.nih.gov/entrez/query.fcgi?cmd=Retrieve&db=pu bmed&dopt=Abstract&list_uids=8136742&query_hl=1

- **Allogeneic bone marrow transplantation for adult acute lymphoblastic leukemia: a single-centre experience.Hematol Oncol.**
  Author(s): Au WY, Lie AK, Ma SK, Chan LC, Lee CK, Kwong YL, Chim CS, Chan TK, Chiu E, Liang R.
  Source: Hematological Oncology.
  http://www.ncbi.nlm.nih.gov/entrez/query.fcgi?cmd=Retrieve&db=pu bmed&dopt=Abstract&list_uids=10414236&query_hl=1

- **Allogeneic bone marrow transplantation in adult acute lymphoblastic leukemia in first complete remission: a comparative study. French Group of Therapy of Adult Acute Lymphoblastic Leukemia.J Clin Oncol.**
  Author(s): Sebban C, Lepage E, Vernant JP, Gluckman E, Attal M, Reiffers J, Sutton L, Racadot E, Michallet M, Maraninchi D, et al.
  Source: Journal of Clinical Oncology : Official Journal of the American Society of Clinical Oncology.
  http://www.ncbi.nlm.nih.gov/entrez/query.fcgi?cmd=Retrieve&db=pu bmed&dopt=Abstract&list_uids=7989932&query_hl=1

- **Alpha-interferon improves survival and remission duration in P-190BCR-ABL positive adult acute lymphoblastic leukemia.Leukemia.**
  Author(s): Visani G, Martinelli G, Piccaluga P, Tosi P, Amabile M, Pastano R, Cavo M, Isidori A, Tura S.
  Source: Leukemia : Official Journal of the Leukemia Society of America, Leukemia Research Fund, U.K.
  http://www.ncbi.nlm.nih.gov/entrez/query.fcgi?cmd=Retrieve&db=pubmed&dopt=Abstract&list_uids=10637472&query_hl=1

- **An extra X chromosome as a sole abnormality in relapse of an adult acute lymphoblastic leukemia.Cancer Genet Cytogenet.**
  Author(s): Yamamoto K, Hato A, Minagawa K, Yakushijin K, Urahama N, Sada A, Okamura A, Ito M, Matsui T.
  Source: Cancer Genetics and Cytogenetics.
  http://www.ncbi.nlm.nih.gov/entrez/query.fcgi?cmd=Retrieve&db=pubmed&dopt=Abstract&list_uids=15571803&query_hl=1

- **Analysis of 20-year follow-up study of LVP regimen for adult acute lymphoblastic leukemia.Int J Hematol.**
  Author(s): Hatta Y, Takeuchi J, Ohshima T, Horikoshi A, Iizuka Y, Kawamura M, Kanemaru M, Horie T.
  Source: International Journal of Hematology.
  http://www.ncbi.nlm.nih.gov/entrez/query.fcgi?cmd=Retrieve&db=pubmed&dopt=Abstract&list_uids=11594516&query_hl=1

- **ATM gene deletion in patients with adult acute lymphoblastic leukemia.Cancer.**
  Author(s): Haidar MA, Kantarjian H, Manshouri T, Chang CY, O'Brien S, Freireich E, Keating M, Albitar M.
  Source: Cancer.
  http://www.ncbi.nlm.nih.gov/entrez/query.fcgi?cmd=Retrieve&db=pubmed&dopt=Abstract&list_uids=10699895&query_hl=1

- **Autologous bone marrow or peripheral blood stem cell transplantation followed by maintenance chemotherapy for adult acute lymphoblastic leukemia in first remission: 50 cases from a single center.Bone Marrow Transplant.**
  Author(s): Powles R, Mehta J, Singhal S, Horton C, Tait D, Milan S, Pollard C, Lumley H, Matthey F, Shirley J, et al.
  Source: Bone Marrow Transplantation.
  http://www.ncbi.nlm.nih.gov/entrez/query.fcgi?cmd=Retrieve&db=pubmed&dopt=Abstract&list_uids=7581142&query_hl=1

- **BCR/ABL translocation in adult acute lymphoblastic leukemia: a comparison of conventional and interphase cytogenetic studies.Cancer Genet Cytogenet.**
  Author(s): So CC, Wong KF, Chung J, Kwong YL.
  Source: Cancer Genetics and Cytogenetics.
  http://www.ncbi.nlm.nih.gov/entrez/query.fcgi?cmd=Retrieve&db=pubmed&dopt=Abstract&list_uids=10198617&query_hl=1

- **Beta-1-integrin expression in adult acute lymphoblastic leukemia: possible relationship with the stem cell antigen CD34.Acta Haematol.**
  Author(s): Cacciola RR, Stagno F, Impera S, Assisi AR, Cacciola E Jr, Guglielmo P.
  Source: Acta Haematologica.
  http://www.ncbi.nlm.nih.gov/entrez/query.fcgi?cmd=Retrieve&db=pubmed&dopt=Abstract&list_uids=8980611&query_hl=1

- **Better outcome of adult acute lymphoblastic leukemia after early genoidentical allogeneic bone marrow transplantation (BMT) than after late high-dose therapy and autologous BMT: a GOELAMS trial.Blood.**
  Author(s): Hunault M, Harousseau JL, Delain M, Truchan-Graczyk M, Cahn JY, Witz F, Lamy T, Pignon B, Jouet JP, Garidi R, Caillot D, Berthou C, Guyotat D, Sadoun A, Sotto JJ, Lioure B, Casassus P, Solal-Celigny P, Stalnikiewicz L, Audhuy B, Blanchet O, Baranger L, Bene MC, Ifrah N; GOELAMS (Groupe Ouest-Est des Leucemies Airgues et Maladies du Sang) Group.
  Source: Blood.
  http://www.ncbi.nlm.nih.gov/entrez/query.fcgi?cmd=Retrieve&db=pubmed&dopt=Abstract&list_uids=15256423&query_hl=1

- **Biology and treatment of adult acute lymphoblastic leukemia.West J Med.**
  Author(s): Levitt L, Lin R.
  Source: The Western Journal of Medicine.
  http://www.ncbi.nlm.nih.gov/entrez/query.fcgi?cmd=Retrieve&db=pubmed&dopt=Abstract&list_uids=8775728&query_hl=1

- **Bolus and continuous infusion mitoxantrone in newly diagnosed adult acute lymphoblastic leukemia: results of two consecutive phase II clinical studies.Cancer Invest.**
  Author(s): Koc Y, Akpek G, Kansu E, Kars A, Tekuzman G, Baltali E, Guler N, Barista I, Gullu I, Ozisik Y, Firat D.
  Source: Cancer Investigation.
  http://www.ncbi.nlm.nih.gov/entrez/query.fcgi?cmd=Retrieve&db=pubmed&dopt=Abstract&list_uids=9679525&query_hl=1

- **Bone marrow biopsy in adult acute lymphoblastic leukemia: morphological characteristics and contribution to the study of prognostic factors.Leuk Res.**
  Author(s): Thomas X, Le QH, Danaila C, Lheritier V, Ffrench M.
  Source: Leukemia Research.
  http://www.ncbi.nlm.nih.gov/entrez/query.fcgi?cmd=Retrieve&db=pubmed&dopt=Abstract&list_uids=12163052&query_hl=1

- **CD34 antigen expression in adult acute lymphoblastic leukemia.Leukemia.**
  Author(s): Kraguljac N, Bogdanovic A, Basara N.
  Source: Leukemia : Official Journal of the Leukemia Society of America, Leukemia Research Fund, U.K.
  http://www.ncbi.nlm.nih.gov/entrez/query.fcgi?cmd=Retrieve&db=pubmed&dopt=Abstract&list_uids=8558931&query_hl=1

- **CD34 expression in adult acute lymphoblastic leukemia.Leuk Lymphoma.**
  Author(s): Cacciola E, Guglielmo P, Cacciola E, Stagno F, Cacciola RR, Impera S.
  Source: Leukemia & Lymphoma.
  http://www.ncbi.nlm.nih.gov/entrez/query.fcgi?cmd=Retrieve&db=pubmed&dopt=Abstract&list_uids=7496352&query_hl=1

- **CD34 expression is associated with major adverse prognostic factors in adult acute lymphoblastic leukemia.Leukemia.**
  Author(s): Thomas X, Archimbaud E, Charrin C, Magaud JP, Fiere D.
  Source: Leukemia : Official Journal of the Leukemia Society of America, Leukemia Research Fund, U.K.
  http://www.ncbi.nlm.nih.gov/entrez/query.fcgi?cmd=Retrieve&db=pubmed&dopt=Abstract&list_uids=7532767&query_hl=1

- **Cell cycle regulatory gene abnormalities are important determinants of leukemogenesis and disease biology in adult acute lymphoblastic leukemia.Blood.**
  Author(s): Stock W, Tsai T, Golden C, Rankin C, Sher D, Slovak ML, Pallavicini MG, Radich JP, Boldt DH.
  Source: Blood.
  http://www.ncbi.nlm.nih.gov/entrez/query.fcgi?cmd=Retrieve&db=pubmed&dopt=Abstract&list_uids=10733508&query_hl=1

- **Change in treatment strategies for adult acute lymphoblastic leukemia (ALL) according to prognostic factors and minimal residual disease.Bone Marrow Transplant.**
  Author(s): Hoelzer D.
  Source: Bone Marrow Transplantation.
  http://www.ncbi.nlm.nih.gov/entrez/query.fcgi?cmd=Retrieve&db=pubmed&dopt=Abstract&list_uids=2390642&query_hl=1

- **Chromosomal abnormalities in adult acute lymphoblastic leukemia: results of the German ALL/AUL Study Group.Recent Results Cancer Res.**
  Author(s): Rieder H, Ludwig WD, Gassmann W, Thiel E, Loffler H, Hoelzer D, Fonatsch C.
  Source: Recent Results in Cancer Research. Fortschritte Der Krebsforschung. Progres Dans Les Recherches Sur Le Cancer.
  http://www.ncbi.nlm.nih.gov/entrez/query.fcgi?cmd=Retrieve&db=pubmed&dopt=Abstract&list_uids=8210634&query_hl=1

- **Clinical and biological importance of cytogenetic abnormalities in childhood and adult acute lymphoblastic leukemia.Ann Med.**
  Author(s): Johansson B, Mertens F, Mitelman F.
  Source: Annals of Medicine.
  http://www.ncbi.nlm.nih.gov/entrez/query.fcgi?cmd=Retrieve&db=pubmed&dopt=Abstract&list_uids=15513300&query_hl=1

- **Clinical importance of myeloid antigen expression in adult acute lymphoblastic leukemia.N Engl J Med.**
  Author(s): Sobol RE, Mick R, Royston I, Davey FR, Ellison RR, Newman R, Cuttner J, Griffin JD, Collins H, Nelson DA, et al.
  Source: The New England Journal of Medicine.
  http://www.ncbi.nlm.nih.gov/entrez/query.fcgi?cmd=Retrieve&db=pubmed&dopt=Abstract&list_uids=3494942&query_hl=1

- **Clinical significance of cytogenetic abnormalities in adult acute lymphoblastic leukemia.Blood.**
  Author(s): Faderl S, Kantarjian HM, Talpaz M, Estrov Z.
  Source: Blood.
  http://www.ncbi.nlm.nih.gov/entrez/query.fcgi?cmd=Retrieve&db=pubmed&dopt=Abstract&list_uids=9596644&query_hl=1

- **Clinical significance of cytogenetic findings at diagnosis and in remission in childhood and adult acute lymphoblastic leukemia: experience from India.Cancer Genet Cytogenet.**
  Author(s): Amare P, Gladstone B, Varghese C, Pai S, Advani S.
  Source: Cancer Genetics and Cytogenetics.
  http://www.ncbi.nlm.nih.gov/entrez/query.fcgi?cmd=Retrieve&db=pubmed&dopt=Abstract&list_uids=10198622&query_hl=1

- **Clinical significance of fragile histidine triad gene expression in adult acute lymphoblastic leukemia.Leuk Res.**
  Author(s): Albitar M, Manshouri T, Gidel C, Croce C, Kornblau S, Pierce S, Kantarjian HM.
  Source: Leukemia Research.
  http://www.ncbi.nlm.nih.gov/entrez/query.fcgi?cmd=Retrieve&db=pubmed&dopt=Abstract&list_uids=11532518&query_hl=1

- **Clinical significance of the BCR-ABL fusion gene in adult acute lymphoblastic leukemia: a Cancer and Leukemia Group B Study (8762).Blood.**
  Author(s): Westbrook CA, Hooberman AL, Spino C, Dodge RK, Larson RA, Davey F, Wurster-Hill DH, Sobol RE, Schiffer C, Bloomfield CD.
  Source: Blood.
  http://www.ncbi.nlm.nih.gov/entrez/query.fcgi?cmd=Retrieve&db=pubmed&dopt=Abstract&list_uids=1467514&query_hl=1

- **Combination chemotherapy of adult acute lymphoblastic leukemia with randomized central nervous system prophylaxis.Blood.**
  Author(s): Omura GA, Moffitt S, Vogler WR, Salter MM.
  Source: Blood.
  http://www.ncbi.nlm.nih.gov/entrez/query.fcgi?cmd=Retrieve&db=pubmed&dopt=Abstract&list_uids=6928104&query_hl=1

- **Comparison of chemotherapy and autologous and allogeneic transplantation as postinduction regimen in adult acute lymphoblastic leukemia: a preliminary multicentric study.Haematol Blood Transfus.**
  Author(s): Fiere D, Broustet A, Leblond V, Maraninchi D, Castaigne S, Flesch M, Varet B, Vernant JP, Milpied N, Troussard X, et al.
  Source: Haematology and Blood Transfusion.
  http://www.ncbi.nlm.nih.gov/entrez/query.fcgi?cmd=Retrieve&db=pubmed&dopt=Abstract&list_uids=2182431&query_hl=1

- **Comparison of the L10M consolidation regimen to an alternative regimen including escalating methotrexate/L-asparaginase for adult acute lymphoblastic leukemia: a Southwest Oncology Group Study.Leukemia.**
  Author(s): Petersdorf SH, Kopecky KJ, Head DR, Boldt DH, Balcerzak SP, Wun T, Roy V, Veith RW, Appelbaum FR.
  Source: Leukemia : Official Journal of the Leukemia Society of America, Leukemia Research Fund, U.K.
  http://www.ncbi.nlm.nih.gov/entrez/query.fcgi?cmd=Retrieve&db=pubmed&dopt=Abstract&list_uids=11236936&query_hl=1

- **Concomitant granulocyte colony-stimulating factor and induction chemoradiotherapy in adult acute lymphoblastic leukemia: a randomized phase III trial.Blood.**
  Author(s): Ottmann OG, Hoelzer D, Gracien E, Ganser A, Kelly K, Reutzel R, Lipp T, Busch FW, Schwonzen M, Heil G, et al.
  Source: Blood.
  http://www.ncbi.nlm.nih.gov/entrez/query.fcgi?cmd=Retrieve&db=pubmed&dopt=Abstract&list_uids=7541660&query_hl=1

- **Consolidation treatment of adult acute lymphoblastic leukemia: a prospective, randomized trial comparing allogeneic versus autologous bone marrow transplantation and testing the impact of recombinant interleukin-2 after autologous bone marrow transplantation. BGMT Group.Blood.**
  Author(s): Attal M, Blaise D, Marit G, Payen C, Michallet M, Vernant JP, Sauvage C, Troussard X, Nedellec G, Pico J, et al.
  Source: Blood.
  http://www.ncbi.nlm.nih.gov/entrez/query.fcgi?cmd=Retrieve&db=pubmed&dopt=Abstract&list_uids=7632972&query_hl=1

- **Cytarabine with high-dose mitoxantrone induces rapid complete remissions in adult acute lymphoblastic leukemia without the use of vincristine or prednisone.J Clin Oncol.**
  Author(s): Weiss M, Maslak P, Feldman E, Berman E, Bertino J, Gee T, Megherian L, Seiter K, Scheinberg D, Golde D.
  Source: Journal of Clinical Oncology : Official Journal of the American Society of Clinical Oncology.
  http://www.ncbi.nlm.nih.gov/entrez/query.fcgi?cmd=Retrieve&db=pu bmed&dopt=Abstract&list_uids=8823326&query_hl=1

- **Cytogenetic analysis of adult acute lymphoblastic leukemia including a Ph+ case surviving more than 5 years.Cancer Genet Cytogenet.**
  Author(s): Fisher TC, Patil SR, Edwards R, Gingrich RD, Burns CP.
  Source: Cancer Genetics and Cytogenetics.
  http://www.ncbi.nlm.nih.gov/entrez/query.fcgi?cmd=Retrieve&db=pu bmed&dopt=Abstract&list_uids=3464344&query_hl=1

- **Cytogenetics and their prognostic value in childhood and adult acute lymphoblastic leukemia (ALL) excluding L3.Hematol Oncol.**
  Author(s): Fenaux P, Lai JL, Morel P, Nelken B, Taboureau O, Deminatti M, Bauters F.
  Source: Hematological Oncology.
  http://www.ncbi.nlm.nih.gov/entrez/query.fcgi?cmd=Retrieve&db=pu bmed&dopt=Abstract&list_uids=2737611&query_hl=1

- **Cytosine arabinoside for induction, salvage, and consolidation therapy of adult acute lymphoblastic leukemia.Semin Oncol.**
  Author(s): Stryckmans P, De Witte T, Bitar N, Marie JP, Suciu S, Solbu G, Debusscher L, Bury J, Peetermans M, Andrien JM, et al.
  Source: Seminars in Oncology.
  http://www.ncbi.nlm.nih.gov/entrez/query.fcgi?cmd=Retrieve&db=pu bmed&dopt=Abstract&list_uids=3296209&query_hl=1

- **der(11)t(1;11)(q11;p15) as an additional cytogenetic abnormality in Ph+ adult acute lymphoblastic leukemia.Cancer Genet Cytogenet.**
  Author(s): Ma SK, Wan TS, Chan LC, Yip SF, Yeung YM.
  Source: Cancer Genetics and Cytogenetics.
  http://www.ncbi.nlm.nih.gov/entrez/query.fcgi?cmd=Retrieve&db=pu bmed&dopt=Abstract&list_uids=10598147&query_hl=1

- **Detection and significance of bcr-abl mRNA transcripts and fusion proteins in Philadelphia-positive adult acute lymphoblastic leukemia.Leukemia.**
  Author(s): Tuszynski A, Dhut S, Young BD, Lister TA, Rohatiner AZ, Amess JA, Chaplin T, Dorey E, Gibbons B.
  Source: Leukemia : Official Journal of the Leukemia Society of America, Leukemia Research Fund, U.K.
  http://www.ncbi.nlm.nih.gov/entrez/query.fcgi?cmd=Retrieve&db=pubmed&dopt=Abstract&list_uids=8412311&query_hl=1

- **Detection of BCR/ABL rearrangements in adult acute lymphoblastic leukemia using a highly sensitive interphase fluorescence in situ hybridization method (D-FISH).Hematol J.**
  Author(s): Mancini M, Nanni M, Sirleto P, De Cuia MR, Castoldi GL, Cilloni D, Cimino G, Mecucci C, Pane F, Annino L, Di Raimondo F, Santoro A, Specchia G, Tedeschi A, Todeschini G, Foa R; GIMEMA study group.
  Source: The Hematology Journal : the Official Journal of the European Haematology Association / Eha.
  http://www.ncbi.nlm.nih.gov/entrez/query.fcgi?cmd=Retrieve&db=pubmed&dopt=Abstract&list_uids=11920234&query_hl=1

- **Detection of BCR-ABL fusion genes in adult acute lymphoblastic leukemia by the polymerase chain reaction.Leukemia.**
  Author(s): Radich JP, Kopecky KJ, Boldt DH, Head D, Slovak ML, Babu R, Kirk J, Lee A, Kessler P, Appelbaum F, et al.
  Source: Leukemia : Official Journal of the Leukemia Society of America, Leukemia Research Fund, U.K.
  http://www.ncbi.nlm.nih.gov/entrez/query.fcgi?cmd=Retrieve&db=pubmed&dopt=Abstract&list_uids=7934164&query_hl=1

- **Detection of MLL gene rearrangements in adult acute lymphoblastic leukemia. A Cancer and Leukemia Group B study.Leukemia.**
  Author(s): Stock W, Thirman MJ, Dodge RK, Rowley JD, Diaz MO, Wurster-Hill D, Sobol RE, Davey FR, Larson RA, Westbrook CA, et al.
  Source: Leukemia : Official Journal of the Leukemia Society of America, Leukemia Research Fund, U.K.
  http://www.ncbi.nlm.nih.gov/entrez/query.fcgi?cmd=Retrieve&db=pubmed&dopt=Abstract&list_uids=7967737&query_hl=1

- **Detection of residual leukemic cells in adult acute lymphoblastic leukemia by analysis of gene rearrangements and correlation with early relapses.Recent Results Cancer Res.**
  Author(s): Knauf WU, Ho AD, Hoelzer D, Thiel E.
  Source: Recent Results in Cancer Research. Fortschritte Der Krebsforschung. Progres Dans Les Recherches Sur Le Cancer.
  http://www.ncbi.nlm.nih.gov/entrez/query.fcgi?cmd=Retrieve&db=pubmed&dopt=Abstract&list_uids=8210639&query_hl=1

- **dic(9;20): a new recurrent chromosome abnormality in adult acute lymphoblastic leukemia.Genes Chromosomes Cancer.**
  Author(s): Rieder H, Schnittger S, Bodenstein H, Schwonzen M, Wormann B, Berkovic D, Ludwig WD, Hoelzer D, Fonatsch C.
  Source: Genes, Chromosomes & Cancer.
  http://www.ncbi.nlm.nih.gov/entrez/query.fcgi?cmd=Retrieve&db=pubmed&dopt=Abstract&list_uids=7541644&query_hl=1

- **Disseminated intravascular coagulation in adult acute lymphoblastic leukemia: frequent complications with fibrinogen levels less than 100 mg/dl.Leuk Lymphoma.**
  Author(s): Sarris A, Cortes J, Kantarjian H, Pierce S, Smith T, Keating M, Koller C, Kornblau S, O'Brien S, Andreeff M.
  Source: Leukemia & Lymphoma.
  http://www.ncbi.nlm.nih.gov/entrez/query.fcgi?cmd=Retrieve&db=pubmed&dopt=Abstract&list_uids=8907274&query_hl=1

- **Dose-intensive therapy for adult acute lymphoblastic leukemia.Semin Oncol.**
  Author(s): Finiewicz KJ, Larson RA.
  Source: Seminars in Oncology.
  http://www.ncbi.nlm.nih.gov/entrez/query.fcgi?cmd=Retrieve&db=pubmed&dopt=Abstract&list_uids=10073558&query_hl=1

- **Early cytoreduction: a major prognostic factor in adult acute lymphoblastic leukemia.Leuk Lymphoma.**
  Author(s): Legrand O, Marie JP, Cadiou M, Blanc C, Ramon S, Zittoun R.
  Source: Leukemia & Lymphoma.
  http://www.ncbi.nlm.nih.gov/entrez/query.fcgi?cmd=Retrieve&db=pubmed&dopt=Abstract&list_uids=7874000&query_hl=1

- **Efficacy of granulocyte and granulocyte-macrophage colony-stimulating factors in the induction treatment of adult acute lymphoblastic leukemia: a multicenter randomized study.Hematol J.**
  Author(s): Thomas X, Boiron JM, Huguet F, Reman O, Sutton L, Turlure P, Garban F, Gardin C, Espinouse D, Boulat O, Lheritier V, Fiere D; Groupe d'Etude et de Traitement de la Leucemie Aigue Lymphoblastique de l'Adulte (GET-LALA Group).
  Source: The Hematology Journal : the Official Journal of the European Haematology Association / Eha.
  http://www.ncbi.nlm.nih.gov/entrez/query.fcgi?cmd=Retrieve&db=pubmed&dopt=Abstract&list_uids=15448664&query_hl=1

- **Estimated 6-year event-free survival of 55% in 60 consecutive adult acute lymphoblastic leukemia patients treated with an intensive phase II protocol based on high induction dose of daunorubicin.Leukemia.**
  Author(s): Todeschini G, Tecchio C, Meneghini V, Pizzolo G, Veneri D, Zanotti R, Ricetti MM, Solero P, April F, Perona G.
  Source: Leukemia : Official Journal of the Leukemia Society of America, Leukemia Research Fund, U.K.
  http://www.ncbi.nlm.nih.gov/entrez/query.fcgi?cmd=Retrieve&db=pubmed&dopt=Abstract&list_uids=9519775&query_hl=1

- **ETV6/AML1 fusion by FISH in adult acute lymphoblastic leukemia.Leukemia.**
  Author(s): Jabber Al-Obaidi MS, Martineau M, Bennett CF, Franklin IM, Goldstone AH, Harewood L, Jalali GR, Prentice HG, Richards SM, Roberts K, Harrison CJ; Medical Research Council Adult Leukaemia Working Party.
  Source: Leukemia : Official Journal of the Leukemia Society of America, Leukemia Research Fund, U.K.
  http://www.ncbi.nlm.nih.gov/entrez/query.fcgi?cmd=Retrieve&db=pubmed&dopt=Abstract&list_uids=11960348&query_hl=1

- **Expression pattern of hybrid phenotype in adult acute lymphoblastic leukemia.Cancer Detect Prev.**
  Author(s): Nakase K, Kita K, Miwa H, Nishii K, Shiku H, Nasu K, Dohy H, Kyo T, Kamada N, Tsutani H.
  Source: Cancer Detection and Prevention.
  http://www.ncbi.nlm.nih.gov/entrez/query.fcgi?cmd=Retrieve&db=pubmed&dopt=Abstract&list_uids=11531016&query_hl=1

- **Expression and long-term prognostic value of CD34 in childhood and adult acute lymphoblastic leukemia.Leuk Lymphoma.**
  Author(s): Vanhaeke DR, Bene MC, Garand R, Faure GC.
  Source: Leukemia & Lymphoma.
  http://www.ncbi.nlm.nih.gov/entrez/query.fcgi?cmd=Retrieve&db=pubmed&dopt=Abstract&list_uids=8750635&query_hl=1

- **Expression of BCL-2 proto-oncogene in adult acute lymphoblastic leukemia.Leukemia.**
  Author(s): Campos L, Sabido O, Sebban C, Charrin C, Bertheas MF, Fiere D, Guyotat D.
  Source: Leukemia : Official Journal of the Leukemia Society of America, Leukemia Research Fund, U.K.
  http://www.ncbi.nlm.nih.gov/entrez/query.fcgi?cmd=Retrieve&db=pubmed&dopt=Abstract&list_uids=8642858&query_hl=1

- **Expression of CD25 (interleukin-2 receptor alpha chain) in adult acute lymphoblastic leukemia predicts for the presence of BCR/ABL fusion transcripts: results of a preliminary laboratory analysis of ECOG/MRC Intergroup Study E2993. Eastern Cooperative Oncology Group/Medical Research Council.Leukemia.**
  Author(s): Paietta E, Racevskis J, Neuberg D, Rowe JM, Goldstone AH, Wiernik PH.
  Source: Leukemia : Official Journal of the Leukemia Society of America, Leukemia Research Fund, U.K.
  http://www.ncbi.nlm.nih.gov/entrez/query.fcgi?cmd=Retrieve&db=pubmed&dopt=Abstract&list_uids=9369422&query_hl=1

- **Expression of the human homologue of rat NG2 in adult acute lymphoblastic leukemia: close association with MLL rearrangement and a CD10(-)/CD24(-)/CD65s(+)/CD15(+) B-cell phenotype.Leukemia.**
  Author(s): Schwartz S, Rieder H, Schlager B, Burmeister T, Fischer L, Thiel E.
  Source: Leukemia : Official Journal of the Leukemia Society of America, Leukemia Research Fund, U.K.
  http://www.ncbi.nlm.nih.gov/entrez/query.fcgi?cmd=Retrieve&db=pubmed&dopt=Abstract&list_uids=12886247&query_hl=1

- **Expression of the multidrug resistance P glycoprotein in newly diagnosed adult acute lymphoblastic leukemia: absence of correlation with response to treatment.Leukemia.**
  Author(s): Wattel E, Lepelley P, Merlat A, Sartiaux C, Bauters F, Jouet JP, Fenaux P.
  Source: Leukemia : Official Journal of the Leukemia Society of America, Leukemia Research Fund, U.K.
  http://www.ncbi.nlm.nih.gov/entrez/query.fcgi?cmd=Retrieve&db=pubmed&dopt=Abstract&list_uids=7475277&query_hl=1

- **Fine characterization of childhood and adult acute lymphoblastic leukemia (ALL) by a proB and preB surrogate light chain-specific mAb and a proposal for a new B cell ALL classification.Leukemia.**
  Author(s): Lemmers B, Arnoulet C, Fossat C, Chambost H, Sainty D, Gabert J, Schiff C.
  Source: Leukemia : Official Journal of the Leukemia Society of America, Leukemia Research Fund, U.K.
  http://www.ncbi.nlm.nih.gov/entrez/query.fcgi?cmd=Retrieve&db=pubmed&dopt=Abstract&list_uids=11187899&query_hl=1

- **Flow-cytometric detection of minimal residual disease in adult acute lymphoblastic leukemia.Haematologica.**
  Author(s): Krampera M, Perbellini O, Maggioni A, Scognamiglio F, Todeschini G, Pizzolo G.
  Source: Haematologica.
  http://www.ncbi.nlm.nih.gov/entrez/query.fcgi?cmd=Retrieve&db=pubmed&dopt=Abstract&list_uids=11255283&query_hl=1

- **Frequency of ETV6/AML1 fusion in adult acute lymphoblastic leukemia.Leukemia.**
  Author(s): Cuneo A, Agostini P, Vitale A, Foa R, Castoldi G.
  Source: Leukemia : Official Journal of the Leukemia Society of America, Leukemia Research Fund, U.K.
  http://www.ncbi.nlm.nih.gov/entrez/query.fcgi?cmd=Retrieve&db=pubmed&dopt=Abstract&list_uids=12592356&query_hl=1

- **Frequent deletions at 12q14.3 chromosomal locus in adult acute lymphoblastic leukemia.Genes Chromosomes Cancer.**
  Author(s): Patel HS, Kantarjian HM, Bueso-Ramos CE, Medeiros LJ, Haidar MA.
  Source: Genes, Chromosomes & Cancer.
  http://www.ncbi.nlm.nih.gov/entrez/query.fcgi?cmd=Retrieve&db=pu
  bmed&dopt=Abstract&list_uids=15495192&query_hl=1

- **G-CSF administered in time-sequenced setting during remission induction and consolidation therapy of adult acute lymphoblastic leukemia has beneficial influence on early recovery and possibly improves long-term outcome: a randomized multicenter study.Leuk Lymphoma.**
  Author(s): Holowiecki J, Giebel S, Krzemien S, Krawczyk-Kulis M, Jagoda K, Kopera M, Holowiecka B, Grosicki S, Hellmann A, Dmoszynska A, Paluszewska M, Robak T, Konopka L, Maj S, Wojnar J, Wojciechowska M, Skotnicki A, Baran W, Cioch M.
  Source: Leukemia & Lymphoma.
  http://www.ncbi.nlm.nih.gov/entrez/query.fcgi?cmd=Retrieve&db=pu
  bmed&dopt=Abstract&list_uids=11999563&query_hl=1

- **GIMEMA ALL - Rescue 97: a salvage strategy for primary refractory or relapsed adult acute lymphoblastic leukemia.Haematologica.**
  Author(s): Camera A, Annino L, Chiurazzi F, Fazi P, Cascavilla N, Fabbiano F, Marmont F, Di Raimondo F, Recchia A, Vignetti M, Rotoli B, Mandelli F.
  Source: Haematologica.
  http://www.ncbi.nlm.nih.gov/entrez/query.fcgi?cmd=Retrieve&db=pu
  bmed&dopt=Abstract&list_uids=15003889&query_hl=1

- **GIMEMA ALL 0288: a multicentric study on adult acute lymphoblastic leukemia. Preliminary results.Leukemia.**
  Author(s): Mandelli F, Annino L, Vegna ML, Camera A, Ciolli S, Deplano W, Fabiano F, Ferrara F, Ladogana S, Muti G, et al.
  Source: Leukemia : Official Journal of the Leukemia Society of America, Leukemia Research Fund, U.K.
  http://www.ncbi.nlm.nih.gov/entrez/query.fcgi?cmd=Retrieve&db=pu
  bmed&dopt=Abstract&list_uids=1578928&query_hl=1

- **Glucocorticoid receptors in adult acute lymphoblastic leukemia.Cancer Res.**
  Author(s): Bloomfield CD, Smith KA, Peterson BA, Munck A.
  Source: Cancer Research.
  http://www.ncbi.nlm.nih.gov/entrez/query.fcgi?cmd=Retrieve&db=pubmed&dopt=Abstract&list_uids=6945909&query_hl=1

- **Granulocyte colony-stimulating factor (G-CSF) as an adjunct to induction chemotherapy of adult acute lymphoblastic leukemia (ALL).Ann Hematol.**
  Author(s): Scherrer R, Geissler K, Kyrle PA, Gisslinger H, Jager U, Bettelheim P, Laczika K, Locker G, Scholten C, Sillaber C, et al.
  Source: Annals of Hematology.
  http://www.ncbi.nlm.nih.gov/entrez/query.fcgi?cmd=Retrieve&db=pubmed&dopt=Abstract&list_uids=7686404&query_hl=1

- **Granulocyte colony-stimulating factor as an adjunct to induction chemotherapy for adult acute lymphoblastic leukemia--a randomized phase-III study.Blood.**
  Author(s): Geissler K, Koller E, Hubmann E, Niederwieser D, Hinterberger W, Geissler D, Kyrle P, Knobl P, Pabinger I, Thalhammer R, Schwarzinger I, Mannhalter C, Jaeger U, Heinz R, Linkesch W, Lechner K.
  Source: Blood.
  http://www.ncbi.nlm.nih.gov/entrez/query.fcgi?cmd=Retrieve&db=pubmed&dopt=Abstract&list_uids=9226158&query_hl=1

- **Hand mirror variant of adult acute lymphoblastic leukemia. Evidence for a mixed leukemia.Am J Clin Pathol.**
  Author(s): Kovarik P, Shrit MA, Yuen B, Radvany R, Schumacher HR.
  Source: American Journal of Clinical Pathology.
  http://www.ncbi.nlm.nih.gov/entrez/query.fcgi?cmd=Retrieve&db=pubmed&dopt=Abstract&list_uids=1283057&query_hl=1

- **Hematopoietic stem cell transplantation in adult acute lymphoblastic leukemia: a single-centre analysis.Leuk Lymphoma.**
  Author(s): Annaloro C, Curioni AC, Molteni M, Della Volpe A, Soligo D, Cortelezzi A, Lambertenghi Deliliers G.
  Source: Leukemia & Lymphoma.
  http://www.ncbi.nlm.nih.gov/entrez/query.fcgi?cmd=Retrieve&db=pubmed&dopt=Abstract&list_uids=15359997&query_hl=1

- **High efficacy of the German multicenter ALL (GMALL) protocol for treatment of adult acute lymphoblastic leukemia (ALL)--a single-institution study.Ann Hematol.**
  Author(s): Scherrer R, Bettelheim P, Geissler K, Jager U, Knobl P, Kyrle PA, Laczika K, Mitterbauer G, Neumann E, Schneider B, et al.
  Source: Annals of Hematology.
  http://www.ncbi.nlm.nih.gov/entrez/query.fcgi?cmd=Retrieve&db=pubmed&dopt=Abstract&list_uids=7948304&query_hl=1

- **High rate of chromosome abnormalities detected by fluorescence in situ hybridization using BCR and ABL probes in adult acute lymphoblastic leukemia.Leukemia.**
  Author(s): Rieder H, Bonwetsch C, Janssen LA, Maurer J, Janssen JW, Schwartz S, Ludwig WD, Gassmann W, Bartram CR, Thiel E, Loffler H, Gokbuget N, Hoelzer D, Fonatsch C.
  Source: Leukemia : Official Journal of the Leukemia Society of America, Leukemia Research Fund, U.K.
  http://www.ncbi.nlm.nih.gov/entrez/query.fcgi?cmd=Retrieve&db=pubmed&dopt=Abstract&list_uids=9737699&query_hl=1

- **High-dose Ara-C plus VM-26 in adult acute lymphoblastic leukemia.Eur J Cancer Clin Oncol.**
  Author(s): Larson RA, Gaynor ER, Shepard KV, Daly KM.
  Source: European Journal of Cancer & Clinical Oncology.
  http://www.ncbi.nlm.nih.gov/entrez/query.fcgi?cmd=Retrieve&db=pubmed&dopt=Abstract&list_uids=3865776&query_hl=1

- **High-dose chemotherapy in adult acute lymphoblastic leukemia.Semin Hematol.**
  Author(s): Hoelzer D.
  Source: Seminars in Hematology.
  http://www.ncbi.nlm.nih.gov/entrez/query.fcgi?cmd=Retrieve&db=pubmed&dopt=Abstract&list_uids=1780759&query_hl=1

- **High-dose methotrexate in the treatment of adult acute lymphoblastic leukemia.Ann Hematol.**
  Author(s): Gokbuget N, Hoelzer D.
  Source: Annals of Hematology.
  http://www.ncbi.nlm.nih.gov/entrez/query.fcgi?cmd=Retrieve&db=pubmed&dopt=Abstract&list_uids=8624372&query_hl=1

- **Hyper-CVAD program in Burkitt's-type adult acute lymphoblastic leukemia.J Clin Oncol.**
  Author(s): Thomas DA, Cortes J, O'Brien S, Pierce S, Faderl S, Albitar M, Hagemeister FB, Cabanillas FF, Murphy S, Keating MJ, Kantarjian H.
  Source: Journal of Clinical Oncology : Official Journal of the American Society of Clinical Oncology.
  http://www.ncbi.nlm.nih.gov/entrez/query.fcgi?cmd=Retrieve&db=pubmed&dopt=Abstract&list_uids=10561310&query_hl=1

- **Immunoglobulin heavy-chain gene rearrangement in adult acute lymphoblastic leukemia reveals preferential usage of J(H)-proximal variable gene segments.Blood.**
  Author(s): Mortuza FY, Moreira IM, Papaioannou M, Gameiro P, Coyle LA, Gricks CS, Amlot P, Prentice HG, Madrigal A, Hoffbrand AV, Foroni L.
  Source: Blood.
  http://www.ncbi.nlm.nih.gov/entrez/query.fcgi?cmd=Retrieve&db=pubmed&dopt=Abstract&list_uids=11313263&query_hl=1

- **Immunophenotype of adult acute lymphoblastic leukemia, clinical parameters, and outcome: an analysis of a prospective trial including 562 tested patients (LALA87). French Group on Therapy for Adult Acute Lymphoblastic Leukemia.Blood.**
  Author(s): Boucheix C, David B, Sebban C, Racadot E, Bene MC, Bernard A, Campos L, Jouault H, Sigaux F, Lepage E, et al.
  Source: Blood.
  http://www.ncbi.nlm.nih.gov/entrez/query.fcgi?cmd=Retrieve&db=pubmed&dopt=Abstract&list_uids=8068949&query_hl=1

- **Immunophenotypes and outcome of Philadelphia chromosome-positive and -negative Thai adult acute lymphoblastic leukemia.Int J Hematol.**
  Author(s): Udomsakdi-Auewarakul C, Promsuwicha O, Tocharoentanaphol C, Munhketvit C, Pattanapanyasat K, Issaragrisil S.
  Source: International Journal of Hematology.
  http://www.ncbi.nlm.nih.gov/entrez/query.fcgi?cmd=Retrieve&db=pubmed&dopt=Abstract&list_uids=14686492&query_hl=1

- **Immunophenotypic aberrancy in adult acute lymphoblastic leukemia.Am J Clin Pathol.**
  Author(s): Ross CW, Stoolman LM, Schnitzer B, Schlegelmilch JA, Hanson CA.
  Source: American Journal of Clinical Pathology.
  http://www.ncbi.nlm.nih.gov/entrez/query.fcgi?cmd=Retrieve&db=pubmed&dopt=Abstract&list_uids=2239822&query_hl=1

- **Immunophenotypic features of childhood and adult acute lymphoblastic leukemia (ALL): experience of the German Multicentre Trials ALL-BFM and GMALL.Leuk Lymphoma.**
  Author(s): Ludwig WD, Reiter A, Loffler H, Gokbuget, Hoelzer D, Riehm H, Thiel E.
  Source: Leukemia & Lymphoma.
  http://www.ncbi.nlm.nih.gov/entrez/query.fcgi?cmd=Retrieve&db=pubmed&dopt=Abstract&list_uids=8075585&query_hl=1

- **Improved results of treatment of adult acute lymphoblastic leukemia.Blood.**
  Author(s): Linker CA, Levitt LJ, O'Donnell M, Ries CA, Link MP, Forman SJ, Farbstein MJ.
  Source: Blood.
  http://www.ncbi.nlm.nih.gov/entrez/query.fcgi?cmd=Retrieve&db=pubmed&dopt=Abstract&list_uids=3470055&query_hl=1

- **Improved survival in adult acute lymphoblastic leukemia. Need for more effective CNS prophylaxis.Am J Clin Oncol.**
  Author(s): Stein RS, Baer MR, Flexner JM.
  Source: American Journal of Clinical Oncology : the Official Publication of the American Radium Society.
  http://www.ncbi.nlm.nih.gov/entrez/query.fcgi?cmd=Retrieve&db=pubmed&dopt=Abstract&list_uids=3869432&query_hl=1

- **Improved treatment outcome in adult acute lymphoblastic leukemia using the intensive German protocol, a preliminary report.Hematol Oncol.**
  Author(s): Chim CS, Kwong YL, Chu YC, Chan CH, Chan YT, Liang R.
  Source: Hematological Oncology.
  http://www.ncbi.nlm.nih.gov/entrez/query.fcgi?cmd=Retrieve&db=pubmed&dopt=Abstract&list_uids=9378468&query_hl=1

- **In vitro culture with prednisolone increases BCL-2 protein expression in adult acute lymphoblastic leukemia cells.Am J Hematol.**
  Author(s): Tosi P, Visani G, Ottaviani E, Manfroi S, Tura S.
  Source: American Journal of Hematology.
  http://www.ncbi.nlm.nih.gov/entrez/query.fcgi?cmd=Retrieve&db=pubmed&dopt=Abstract&list_uids=8602624&query_hl=1

- **In vitro depletion of clonogenic cells in adult acute lymphoblastic leukemia with a CD10 (anti-cALLA) monoclonal antibody.Eur J Cancer Clin Oncol.**
  Author(s): Marie JP, Choquet C, Perrot JY, Thevenin D, Pillier C, Boucheix C, Zittoun R.
  Source: European Journal of Cancer & Clinical Oncology.
  http://www.ncbi.nlm.nih.gov/entrez/query.fcgi?cmd=Retrieve&db=pubmed&dopt=Abstract&list_uids=3308484&query_hl=1

- **In vitro drug resistance profiles of adult acute lymphoblastic leukemia: possible explanation for difference in outcome to similar therapeutic regimens.Leuk Lymphoma.**
  Author(s): Styczynski J, Wysocki M.
  Source: Leukemia & Lymphoma.
  http://www.ncbi.nlm.nih.gov/entrez/query.fcgi?cmd=Retrieve&db=pubmed&dopt=Abstract&list_uids=11999561&query_hl=1

- **Increasing risk of relapse after allogeneic stem cell transplant for adult acute lymphoblastic leukemia in > or = 2nd complete remission induced by highly intensive chemotherapy.Haematologica.**
  Author(s): Mengarelli A, Iori AP, Cerretti R, Cerilli L, Romano A, Arcese W.
  Source: Haematologica.
  http://www.ncbi.nlm.nih.gov/entrez/query.fcgi?cmd=Retrieve&db=pubmed&dopt=Abstract&list_uids=12091136&query_hl=1

- **Induction therapy by frequent administration of doxorubicin with four other drugs, followed by intensive consolidation and maintenance therapy for adult acute lymphoblastic leukemia: the JALSG-ALL93 study.Leukemia.**
  Author(s): Takeuchi J, Kyo T, Naito K, Sao H, Takahashi M, Miyawaki S, Kuriyama K, Ohtake S, Yagasaki F, Murakami H, Asou N, Ino T, Okamoto T, Usui N, Nishimura M, Shinagawa K, Fukushima T, Taguchi H, Morii T, Mizuta S, Akiyama H, Nakamura Y, Ohshima T, Ohno R.
  Source: Leukemia : Official Journal of the Leukemia Society of America, Leukemia Research Fund, U.K.
  http://www.ncbi.nlm.nih.gov/entrez/query.fcgi?cmd=Retrieve&db=pubmed&dopt=Abstract&list_uids=12094249&query_hl=1

- **Infectious complications in adult acute lymphoblastic leukemia (ALL): experience at one single center.Leuk Lymphoma.**
  Author(s): Offidani M, Corvatta L, Malerba L, Marconi M, Leoni P.
  Source: Leukemia & Lymphoma.
  http://www.ncbi.nlm.nih.gov/entrez/query.fcgi?cmd=Retrieve&db=pubmed&dopt=Abstract&list_uids=15370214&query_hl=1

- **Insertion of chromosome 11 in chromosome 4 resulting in a 5'MLL-3'AF4 fusion gene in a case of adult acute lymphoblastic leukemia.Cancer Genet Cytogenet.**
  Author(s): Morel F, Le Bris MJ, Douet-Guilbert N, Duchemin J, Herry A, Le Calvez G, Marion V, Berthou C, De Braekeleer M.
  Source: Cancer Genetics and Cytogenetics.
  http://www.ncbi.nlm.nih.gov/entrez/query.fcgi?cmd=Retrieve&db=pubmed&dopt=Abstract&list_uids=12885467&query_hl=1

- **Intensified and shortened cyclical chemotherapy for adult acute lymphoblastic leukemia.J Clin Oncol.**
  Author(s): Linker C, Damon L, Ries C, Navarro W.
  Source: Journal of Clinical Oncology : Official Journal of the American Society of Clinical Oncology.
  http://www.ncbi.nlm.nih.gov/entrez/query.fcgi?cmd=Retrieve&db=pubmed&dopt=Abstract&list_uids=12011123&query_hl=1

- **Intensive salvage chemotherapy for primary refractory or first relapsed adult acute lymphoblastic leukemia: results of a prospective trial.Haematologica.**
  Author(s): Martino R, Bellido M, Brunet S, Altes A, Sureda A, Guardia R, Aventin A, Nomdedeu JF, Domingo-Albos A, Sierra J.
  Source: Haematologica.
  http://www.ncbi.nlm.nih.gov/entrez/query.fcgi?cmd=Retrieve&db=pubmed&dopt=Abstract&list_uids=10366793&query_hl=1

- **Intensive therapy before or during the conditioning regimen of allogeneic marrow transplantation in adult acute lymphoblastic leukemia patients: we must choose to reduce Toxicity--a Groupe Ouest-Est d'Etude des Leucemies et Autres Maladies du Sang study.Biol Blood Marrow Transplant.**
  Author(s): Deconinck E, Hunault M, Milpied N, Bernard M, Renaud M, Desablens B, Delain M, Witz F, Lioure B, Pignon B, Guyotat D, Berthou C, Jouet JP, Casassus P, Ifrah N, Boiron JM.
  Source: Biology of Blood and Marrow Transplantation : Journal of the American Society for Blood and Marrow Transplantation.
  http://www.ncbi.nlm.nih.gov/entrez/query.fcgi?cmd=Retrieve&db=pubmed&dopt=Abstract&list_uids=15931633&query_hl=1

- **Intensive therapy for adult acute lymphoblastic leukemia.Semin Hematol.**
  Author(s): Berman E, Weiss M, Kempin S, Gee T, Bertino J, Clarkson B.
  Source: Seminars in Hematology.
  http://www.ncbi.nlm.nih.gov/entrez/query.fcgi?cmd=Retrieve&db=pubmed&dopt=Abstract&list_uids=1780756&query_hl=1

- **Intensive therapy for adult acute lymphoblastic leukemia: preliminary results of the idarubicin/vincristine/L-asparaginase/prednisolone regimen.Semin Oncol.**
  Author(s): Bassan R, Battista R, Viero P, Pogliani E, Rossi G, Lambertenghi-Deliliers G, Rambaldi A, D'Emilio A, Buelli M, Borleri G, et al.
  Source: Seminars in Oncology.
  http://www.ncbi.nlm.nih.gov/entrez/query.fcgi?cmd=Retrieve&db=pubmed&dopt=Abstract&list_uids=7507263&query_hl=1

- **In-vitro granulopoiesis in adult acute lymphoblastic leukemia at various phases of the disease.Leuk Res.**
  Author(s): Shih LY, Chiu WF.
  Source: Leukemia Research.
  http://www.ncbi.nlm.nih.gov/entrez/query.fcgi?cmd=Retrieve&db=pubmed&dopt=Abstract&list_uids=3472014&query_hl=1

- **Is the scoring system an effective clinico-biological tool in myeloid antigen positive adult acute lymphoblastic leukemia? Results of a long-term study.Hematol J.**
  Author(s): Cascavilla N, Musto P, Melillo L, Bodenizza C, Dell'Olio M, Nobile M, Minervini MM, Perla G, D'Arena G, Carella AM.
  Source: The Hematology Journal : the Official Journal of the European Haematology Association / Eha.
  http://www.ncbi.nlm.nih.gov/entrez/query.fcgi?cmd=Retrieve&db=pubmed&dopt=Abstract&list_uids=12391543&query_hl=1

- **Lack of CpG island methylator phenotype defines a clinical subtype of T-cell acute lymphoblastic leukemia associated with good prognosis.J Clin Oncol.**
  Author(s): Roman-Gomez J, Jimenez-Velasco A, Agirre X, Prosper F, Heiniger A, Torres A.
  Source: Journal of Clinical Oncology : Official Journal of the American Society of Clinical Oncology.
  http://www.ncbi.nlm.nih.gov/entrez/query.fcgi?cmd=Retrieve&db=pubmed&dopt=Abstract&list_uids=16192589&query_hl=2

- **Late intensification chemotherapy has not improved the results of intensive chemotherapy in adult acute lymphoblastic leukemia. Results of a prospective multicenter randomized trial (PETHEMA ALL-89). Spanish Society of Hematology.Haematologica.**
  Author(s): Ribera JM, Ortega JJ, Oriol A, Fontanillas M, Hernandez-Rivas JM, Brunet S, Garcia-Conde J, Maldonado J, Zuazu J, Gardella S, Besalduch J, Leon P, Macia J, Domingo-Albos A, Feliu E, San Miguel JF.
  Source: Haematologica.
  http://www.ncbi.nlm.nih.gov/entrez/query.fcgi?cmd=Retrieve&db=pubmed&dopt=Abstract&list_uids=9573676&query_hl=1

- **Lithium and granulocytopenia during induction treatment of adult acute lymphoblastic leukemia.Tumori.**
  Author(s): Bandini G, Ricci P, Ruggero D, Cantore M, Visani G, Tura S.
  Source: Tumori.
  http://www.ncbi.nlm.nih.gov/entrez/query.fcgi?cmd=Retrieve&db=pu
  bmed&dopt=Abstract&list_uids=6960590&query_hl=1

- **Long term survivors in adult acute lymphoblastic leukemia.Bone Marrow Transplant.**
  Author(s): Tura S, Visani G.
  Source: Bone Marrow Transplantation.
  http://www.ncbi.nlm.nih.gov/entrez/query.fcgi?cmd=Retrieve&db=pu
  bmed&dopt=Abstract&list_uids=2653481&query_hl=1

- **Long-term follow-up of intensive ara-C-based chemotherapy followed by bone marrow transplantation for adult acute lymphoblastic leukemia: impact of induction Ara-C dose and post-remission therapy.Leuk Res.**
  Author(s): Sotomayor EM, Piantadosi S, Miller CB, Karp JE, Jones RJ, Rowley SD, Kaufmann SH, Braine H, Burke PJ, Gore SD.
  Source: Leukemia Research.
  http://www.ncbi.nlm.nih.gov/entrez/query.fcgi?cmd=Retrieve&db=pu
  bmed&dopt=Abstract&list_uids=11916520&query_hl=1

- **Long-term follow-up of patients with newly diagnosed adult acute lymphoblastic leukemia: a single institution experience of 378 consecutive patients over a 21-year period.Leukemia.**
  Author(s): Thomas X, Danaila C, Le QH, Sebban C, Troncy J, Charrin C, Lheritier V, Michallet M, Magaud JP, Fiere D.
  Source: Leukemia : Official Journal of the Leukemia Society of America, Leukemia Research Fund, U.K.
  http://www.ncbi.nlm.nih.gov/entrez/query.fcgi?cmd=Retrieve&db=pu
  bmed&dopt=Abstract&list_uids=11753600&query_hl=1

- **Long-term relapse-free survival in adult acute lymphoblastic leukemia.Cancer Treat Rep.**
  Author(s): Gingrich RD, Burns CP, Armitage JO, Aunan SB, Edwards RW, Dick FR, Maguire LC, Leimert JT.
  Source: Cancer Treatment Reports.
  http://www.ncbi.nlm.nih.gov/entrez/query.fcgi?cmd=Retrieve&db=pu
  bmed&dopt=Abstract&list_uids=3855697&query_hl=1

- **Long-term results of autologous bone marrow transplantation in adult acute lymphoblastic leukemia.Leuk Lymphoma.**
  Author(s): Lambertenghi Deliliers G, Mozzana R, Annaloro C, Butti C, Della Volpe A, Oriani A, Pozzoli E, Soligo D, Polli EE.
  Source: Leukemia & Lymphoma.
  http://www.ncbi.nlm.nih.gov/entrez/query.fcgi?cmd=Retrieve&db=pubmed&dopt=Abstract&list_uids=8124215&query_hl=1

- **Long-term survival in adolescent and adult acute lymphoblastic leukemia.Cancer.**
  Author(s): Amadori S, Meloni G, Baccarani M, Haanen C, Willemze R, Corbelli G, Drenthe-Schonk A, Cardozo PL, Tura S, Mandelli F.
  Source: Cancer.
  http://www.ncbi.nlm.nih.gov/entrez/query.fcgi?cmd=Retrieve&db=pubmed&dopt=Abstract&list_uids=6573940&query_hl=1

- **Long-term survival in adult acute lymphoblastic leukemia: follow-up of a Southeastern Cancer Study Group trial.J Clin Oncol.**
  Author(s): Omura GA, Raney M.
  Source: Journal of Clinical Oncology : Official Journal of the American Society of Clinical Oncology.
  http://www.ncbi.nlm.nih.gov/entrez/query.fcgi?cmd=Retrieve&db=pubmed&dopt=Abstract&list_uids=3860630&query_hl=1

- **Low frequency of TEL/AML1 in adult acute lymphoblastic leukemia.Cancer Genet Cytogenet.**
  Author(s): Kwong YL, Wong KF.
  Source: Cancer Genetics and Cytogenetics.
  http://www.ncbi.nlm.nih.gov/entrez/query.fcgi?cmd=Retrieve&db=pubmed&dopt=Abstract&list_uids=9332479&query_hl=1

- **Management of adult acute lymphoblastic leukemia: moving toward a risk-adapted approach.Curr Opin Oncol.**
  Author(s): Verma A, Stock W.
  Source: Current Opinion in Oncology.
  http://www.ncbi.nlm.nih.gov/entrez/query.fcgi?cmd=Retrieve&db=pubmed&dopt=Abstract&list_uids=11148680&query_hl=1

- **MDR1 protein expression is an independent predictor of complete remission in newly diagnosed adult acute lymphoblastic leukemia.Blood.**
  Author(s): Tafuri A, Gregorj C, Petrucci MT, Ricciardi MR, Mancini M, Cimino G, Mecucci C, Tedeschi A, Fioritoni G, Ferrara F, Di Raimondo F, Gallo E, Liso V, Fabbiano F, Cascavilla N, Pizzolo G, Camera A, Pane F, Lanza F, Cilloni D, Annino L, Vitale A, Vegna ML, Vignetti M, Foa R, Mandelli F; GIMEMA Group.
  Source: Blood.
  http://www.ncbi.nlm.nih.gov/entrez/query.fcgi?cmd=Retrieve&db=pubmed&dopt=Abstract&list_uids=12130511&query_hl=1

- **Minimal residual disease tests provide an independent predictor of clinical outcome in adult acute lymphoblastic leukemia.J Clin Oncol.**
  Author(s): Mortuza FY, Papaioannou M, Moreira IM, Coyle LA, Gameiro P, Gandini D, Prentice HG, Goldstone A, Hoffbrand AV, Foroni L.
  Source: Journal of Clinical Oncology : Official Journal of the American Society of Clinical Oncology.
  http://www.ncbi.nlm.nih.gov/entrez/query.fcgi?cmd=Retrieve&db=pubmed&dopt=Abstract&list_uids=11844835&query_hl=1

- **Molecular cytogenetic study of instability at 1q21 approximately q32 in adult acute lymphoblastic leukemia.Cancer Genet Cytogenet.**
  Author(s): Specchia G, Albano F, Anelli L, Zagaria A, Liso A, Pannunzio A, Archidiacono N, Liso V, Rocchi M.
  Source: Cancer Genetics and Cytogenetics.
  http://www.ncbi.nlm.nih.gov/entrez/query.fcgi?cmd=Retrieve&db=pubmed&dopt=Abstract&list_uids=15588856&query_hl=1

- **Molecular genetic events in adult acute lymphoblastic leukemia.Expert Rev Mol Diagn.**
  Author(s): Gleissner B, Thiel E.
  Source: Expert Review of Molecular Diagnostics.
  http://www.ncbi.nlm.nih.gov/entrez/query.fcgi?cmd=Retrieve&db=pubmed&dopt=Abstract&list_uids=12779008&query_hl=1

- **MR findings in Balint's syndrome, following intrathecal methotrexate and cytarabine therapy in adult acute lymphoblastic leukemia.Eur Neurol.**
  Author(s): Hollinger P, Zenhausern R, Schroth G, Mattle HP.
  Source: European Neurology.
  http://www.ncbi.nlm.nih.gov/entrez/query.fcgi?cmd=Retrieve&db=pubmed&dopt=Abstract&list_uids=11598342&query_hl=1

- **Multiple bone lesions after allogeneic bone marrow transplantation in a patient with relapsed adult acute lymphoblastic leukemia: minimal residual disease analysis may predict extramedullary relapse.Leuk Lymphoma.**
  Author(s): Nomura K, Okamoto T, Nakao M, Ueda K, Akano Y, Fujita Y, Kobayashi M, Yokota S, Horiike S, Nishida K, Kusuzaki K, Taniwaki M.
  Source: Leukemia & Lymphoma.
  http://www.ncbi.nlm.nih.gov/entrez/query.fcgi?cmd=Retrieve&db=pubmed&dopt=Abstract&list_uids=11911412&query_hl=1

- **Myeloid antigen expression in adult acute lymphoblastic leukemia: clinicohematological correlations and prognostic relevance.Hematol Pathol.**
  Author(s): Ferrara F, De Rosa C, Fasanaro A, Mele G, Finizio O, Schiavone EM, Spada OA, Rametta V, Del Vecchio L.
  Source: Hematologic Pathology.
  http://www.ncbi.nlm.nih.gov/entrez/query.fcgi?cmd=Retrieve&db=pubmed&dopt=Abstract&list_uids=2373674&query_hl=1

- **Myeloid antigen expression provides favorable outcome in patients with adult acute lymphoblastic leukemia: a single-center study.Ann Hematol.**
  Author(s): Yenerel MN, Atamer T, Yavuz AS, Kucukkaya R, Besisik S, Aktan M, Keskin H, Nalcaci M, Sargin D, Pekcelen Y, Dincol G.
  Source: Annals of Hematology.
  http://www.ncbi.nlm.nih.gov/entrez/query.fcgi?cmd=Retrieve&db=pubmed&dopt=Abstract&list_uids=12373349&query_hl=1

- **Myeloid surface antigen expression in adult acute lymphoblastic leukemia.Leukemia.**
  Author(s): Guyotat D, Campos L, Shi ZH, Charrin C, Treille D, Magaud JP, Fiere D.
  Source: Leukemia : Official Journal of the Leukemia Society of America, Leukemia Research Fund, U.K.
  http://www.ncbi.nlm.nih.gov/entrez/query.fcgi?cmd=Retrieve&db=pu bmed&dopt=Abstract&list_uids=1697640&query_hl=1

- **Myeloid-antigen expression in adult acute lymphoblastic leukemia.N Engl J Med.**
  Author(s): Drexler HG.
  Source: The New England Journal of Medicine.
  http://www.ncbi.nlm.nih.gov/entrez/query.fcgi?cmd=Retrieve&db=pu bmed&dopt=Abstract&list_uids=3477697&query_hl=1

- **Myeloperoxidase immunoreactivity in adult acute lymphoblastic leukemia.Am J Clin Pathol.**
  Author(s): Arber DA, Snyder DS, Fine M, Dagis A, Niland J, Slovak ML.
  Source: American Journal of Clinical Pathology.
  http://www.ncbi.nlm.nih.gov/entrez/query.fcgi?cmd=Retrieve&db=pu bmed&dopt=Abstract&list_uids=11447748&query_hl=1

- **Nation-wide randomized comparative study of doxorubicin, vincristine and prednisolone combination therapy with and without L-asparaginase for adult acute lymphoblastic leukemia.Cancer Chemother Pharmacol.**
  Author(s): Nagura E, Kimura K, Yamada K, Ota K, Maekawa T, Takaku F, Uchino H, Masaoka T, Amaki I, Kawashima K, et al.
  Source: Cancer Chemotherapy and Pharmacology.
  http://www.ncbi.nlm.nih.gov/entrez/query.fcgi?cmd=Retrieve&db=pu bmed&dopt=Abstract&list_uids=8306408&query_hl=1

- **Non-myeloablative conditioning before allogeneic stem cell transplantation in adult acute lymphoblastic leukemia.Haematologica.**
  Author(s): Gokbuget N, Hoelzer D.
  Source: Haematologica.
  http://www.ncbi.nlm.nih.gov/entrez/query.fcgi?cmd=Retrieve&db=pu bmed&dopt=Abstract&list_uids=12745266&query_hl=1

- **Outcome of adult acute lymphoblastic leukemia: a single center experience.J Pak Med Assoc.**
  Author(s): Usman M, Burney I, Nasim A, Adil SN, Salam A, Siddiqui T, Khurshid M.
  Source: Jpma. the Journal of the Pakistan Medical Association.
  http://www.ncbi.nlm.nih.gov/entrez/query.fcgi?cmd=Retrieve&db=pubmed&dopt=Abstract&list_uids=14620310&query_hl=1

- **Outcome of Philadelphia chromosome-positive adult acute lymphoblastic leukemia.Leuk Lymphoma.**
  Author(s): Faderl S, Kantarjian HM, Thomas DA, Cortes J, Giles F, Pierce S, Albitar M, Estrov Z.
  Source: Leukemia & Lymphoma.
  http://www.ncbi.nlm.nih.gov/entrez/query.fcgi?cmd=Retrieve&db=pubmed&dopt=Abstract&list_uids=10674898&query_hl=1

- **Outcome of treatment in adult acute lymphoblastic leukemia in southern Brazil using a modified german multicenter acute lymphoblastic leukemia protocol.Acta Haematol.**
  Author(s): Fogliatto L, Bittencourt H, Nunes AS, Salenave PR, Silva GS, Daudt LE, Job FM, Bittencourt R, Onsten T, Silla LM.
  Source: Acta Haematologica.
  http://www.ncbi.nlm.nih.gov/entrez/query.fcgi?cmd=Retrieve&db=pubmed&dopt=Abstract&list_uids=12053147&query_hl=1

- **Partial deletions of long arm of chromosome 6: biologic and clinical implications in adult acute lymphoblastic leukemia.Leukemia.**
  Author(s): Mancini M, Vegna ML, Castoldi GL, Mecucci C, Spirito F, Elia L, Tafuri A, Annino L, Pane F, Rege-Cambrin G, Gottardi M, Leoni P, Gallo E, Camera A, Luciano L, Specchia G, Torelli G, Sborgia M, Gabbas A, Tedeschi A, Della Starza I, Cascavilla N, Di Raimondo F, Mandelli F, Foa R.
  Source: Leukemia : Official Journal of the Leukemia Society of America, Leukemia Research Fund, U.K.
  http://www.ncbi.nlm.nih.gov/entrez/query.fcgi?cmd=Retrieve&db=pubmed&dopt=Abstract&list_uids=12357357&query_hl=1

- **Persistence of peripheral blood and bone marrow blasts during remission induction in adult acute lymphoblastic leukemia confers a poor prognosis depending on treatment intensity.Clin Cancer Res.**
  Author(s): Cortes J, Fayad L, O'Brien S, Keating M, Kantarjian H.
  Source: Clinical Cancer Research : an Official Journal of the American Association for Cancer Research.
  http://www.ncbi.nlm.nih.gov/entrez/query.fcgi?cmd=Retrieve&db=pubmed&dopt=Abstract&list_uids=10499624&query_hl=1

- **Phase II study of etoposide, ifosfamide, and mitoxantrone for the treatment of resistant adult acute lymphoblastic leukemia.Am J Hematol.**
  Author(s): Schiller G, Lee M, Territo M, Gajewski J, Nimer S.
  Source: American Journal of Hematology.
  http://www.ncbi.nlm.nih.gov/entrez/query.fcgi?cmd=Retrieve&db=pubmed&dopt=Abstract&list_uids=8352235&query_hl=1

- **Philadelphia chromosome positive adult acute lymphoblastic leukemia: characteristics, prognostic factors and treatment outcome.Hematol Cell Ther.**
  Author(s): Thomas X, Thiebaut A, Olteanu N, Danaila C, Charrin C, Archimbaud E, Fiere D.
  Source: Hematology and Cell Therapy.
  http://www.ncbi.nlm.nih.gov/entrez/query.fcgi?cmd=Retrieve&db=pubmed&dopt=Abstract&list_uids=9698220&query_hl=1

- **Philadelphia chromosome-positive adult acute lymphoblastic leukemia. Serial chromosome studies in 5 patients.Haematologica.**
  Author(s): Zaccaria A, Rosti G, Testoni N, Gobbi M, Lauria F, Tura S.
  Source: Haematologica.
  http://www.ncbi.nlm.nih.gov/entrez/query.fcgi?cmd=Retrieve&db=pubmed&dopt=Abstract&list_uids=6432641&query_hl=1

- **Philadelphia negative, BCR-ABL positive adult acute lymphoblastic leukemia (ALL) in 2 of 39 patients with combined cytogenetic and molecular analysis.Leukemia.**
  Author(s): Preudhomme C, Fenaux P, Lal JL, Lepelley P, Sartiaux C, Collyn-d'Hooghe M, Zandecki M, Cosson A, Jouet JP, Kerckaert JP.
  Source: Leukemia : Official Journal of the Leukemia Society of America, Leukemia Research Fund, U.K.
  http://www.ncbi.nlm.nih.gov/entrez/query.fcgi?cmd=Retrieve&db=pubmed&dopt=Abstract&list_uids=8321020&query_hl=1

- **Poor outcome of intensive chemotherapy for adult acute lymphoblastic leukemia: a possible dose effect.Leukemia.**
  Author(s): Chiu EK, Chan LC, Liang R, Lie A, Kwong YL, Todd D, Chan TK.
  Source: Leukemia : Official Journal of the Leukemia Society of America, Leukemia Research Fund, U.K.
  http://www.ncbi.nlm.nih.gov/entrez/query.fcgi?cmd=Retrieve&db=pubmed&dopt=Abstract&list_uids=8090027&query_hl=1

- **Population-based study of the pattern of molecular markers of minimal residual disease in childhood and adult acute lymphoblastic leukemia: an assessment of the practical difficulty of representative sampling for trial purposes. Northern Region Haematology Group.Med Pediatr Oncol.**
  Author(s): Middleton PG, Norden J, Levett D, Levasseur M, Miller S, Irving JA, Wood A, Reid MM, Taylor PR, Proctor SJ.
  Source: Medical and Pediatric Oncology.
  http://www.ncbi.nlm.nih.gov/entrez/query.fcgi?cmd=Retrieve&db=pubmed&dopt=Abstract&list_uids=10657870&query_hl=1

- **Predictive factors for outcome of allogeneic hematopoietic cell transplantation for adult acute lymphoblastic leukemia.Biol Blood Marrow Transplant.**
  Author(s): Doney K, Hagglund H, Leisenring W, Chauncey T, Appelbaum FR, Storb R.
  Source: Biology of Blood and Marrow Transplantation : Journal of the American Society for Blood and Marrow Transplantation.
  http://www.ncbi.nlm.nih.gov/entrez/query.fcgi?cmd=Retrieve&db=pubmed&dopt=Abstract&list_uids=12869961&query_hl=1

- **Preleukemic state preceding adult acute lymphoblastic leukemia.Am J Med.**
  Author(s): Dayton MA, van Besien K, Tricot G, Hoffman R.
  Source: The American Journal of Medicine.
  http://www.ncbi.nlm.nih.gov/entrez/query.fcgi?cmd=Retrieve&db=pubmed&dopt=Abstract&list_uids=2239985&query_hl=1

- **Prethymic phenotype and genotype of pre-T (CD7+/ER-)-cell leukemia and its clinical significance within adult acute lymphoblastic leukemia.Blood.**
  Author(s): Thiel E, Kranz BR, Raghavachar A, Bartram CR, Loffler H, Messerer D, Ganser A, Ludwig WD, Buchner T, Hoelzer D.
  Source: Blood.
  http://www.ncbi.nlm.nih.gov/entrez/query.fcgi?cmd=Retrieve&db=pubmed&dopt=Abstract&list_uids=2467704&query_hl=1

- **Primary refractory and relapsed adult acute lymphoblastic leukemia: characteristics, treatment results, and prognosis with salvage therapy.Cancer.**
  Author(s): Thomas DA, Kantarjian H, Smith TL, Koller C, Cortes J, O'Brien S, Giles FJ, Gajewski J, Pierce S, Keating MJ.
  Source: Cancer.
  http://www.ncbi.nlm.nih.gov/entrez/query.fcgi?cmd=Retrieve&db=pubmed&dopt=Abstract&list_uids=10506707&query_hl=1

- **Prognostic factor analysis of central nervous system relapse in adult acute lymphoblastic leukemia. A Southeastern Cancer Study Group report.Am J Clin Oncol.**
  Author(s): Omura GA, Bass D.
  Source: American Journal of Clinical Oncology : the Official Publication of the American Radium Society.
  http://www.ncbi.nlm.nih.gov/entrez/query.fcgi?cmd=Retrieve&db=pubmed&dopt=Abstract&list_uids=8141113&query_hl=1

- **Prognostic factors and outcome of therapy in adult acute lymphoblastic leukemia.Indian J Cancer.**
  Author(s): Philips GK, Crowell EB Jr, Mani A.
  Source: Indian Journal of Cancer.
  http://www.ncbi.nlm.nih.gov/entrez/query.fcgi?cmd=Retrieve&db=pubmed&dopt=Abstract&list_uids=1786981&query_hl=1

- **Prognostic factors in adult acute lymphoblastic leukemia (ALL).Bone Marrow Transplant.**
  Author(s): Mazzucconi MG, Amadori S, Mandelli F.
  Source: Bone Marrow Transplantation.
  http://www.ncbi.nlm.nih.gov/entrez/query.fcgi?cmd=Retrieve&db=pubmed&dopt=Abstract&list_uids=2713566&query_hl=1

- **Prognostic factors in adult acute lymphoblastic leukemia.Haematol Blood Transfus.**
  Author(s): Lister TA, Roberts MM, Brearley RL, Cullen MH, Greaves MF.
  Source: Haematology and Blood Transfusion.
  http://www.ncbi.nlm.nih.gov/entrez/query.fcgi?cmd=Retrieve&db=pubmed&dopt=Abstract&list_uids=296119&query_hl=1

- **Prognostic factors in adult acute lymphoblastic leukemia.Hematology.**
  Author(s): Thomas X, Le QH.
  Source: Hematology (Amsterdam, Netherlands)
  http://www.ncbi.nlm.nih.gov/entrez/query.fcgi?cmd=Retrieve&db=pubmed&dopt=Abstract&list_uids=12911941&query_hl=1

- **Prognostic importance of immunologic markers in adult acute lymphoblastic leukemia.N Engl J Med.**
  Author(s): Greaves MF, Lister TA.
  Source: The New England Journal of Medicine.
  http://www.ncbi.nlm.nih.gov/entrez/query.fcgi?cmd=Retrieve&db=pubmed&dopt=Abstract&list_uids=6934374&query_hl=1

- **Prognostic influence of pretreatment characteristics in adult acute lymphoblastic leukemia.Blood.**
  Author(s): Leimert JT, Burns CP, Wiltse CG, Armitage JO, Clarke WR.
  Source: Blood.
  http://www.ncbi.nlm.nih.gov/entrez/query.fcgi?cmd=Retrieve&db=pubmed&dopt=Abstract&list_uids=6931623&query_hl=1

- **Prognostic value of early response to chemotherapy assessed by the day 15 bone marrow aspiration in adult acute lymphoblastic leukemia: a prospective analysis of 437 cases and its application for designing induction chemotherapy trials.Leuk Res.**
  Author(s): Sebban C, Browman GP, Lepage E, Fiere D.
  Source: Leukemia Research.
  http://www.ncbi.nlm.nih.gov/entrez/query.fcgi?cmd=Retrieve&db=pubmed&dopt=Abstract&list_uids=8551804&query_hl=1

- **Prognostic value of the rapidity of bone marrow blast cell proliferation in adult acute lymphoblastic leukemia.Leukemia.**
  Author(s): Pich A, Chiusa L, Ceretto C, Fornari A, Audisio E, Marmont F, Navone R.
  Source: Leukemia : Official Journal of the Leukemia Society of America, Leukemia Research Fund, U.K.
  http://www.ncbi.nlm.nih.gov/entrez/query.fcgi?cmd=Retrieve&db=pubmed&dopt=Abstract&list_uids=14586475&query_hl=1

- **Progress and challenges in the therapy of adult acute lymphoblastic leukemia.Curr Opin Hematol.**
  Author(s): Kebriaei P, Larson RA.
  Source: Current Opinion in Hematology.
  http://www.ncbi.nlm.nih.gov/entrez/query.fcgi?cmd=Retrieve&db=pubmed&dopt=Abstract&list_uids=12799534&query_hl=1

- **Progress in adult acute lymphoblastic leukemia.West J Med.**
  Author(s): Appelbaum FR.
  Source: The Western Journal of Medicine.
  http://www.ncbi.nlm.nih.gov/entrez/query.fcgi?cmd=Retrieve&db=pubmed&dopt=Abstract&list_uids=8775741&query_hl=1

- **Prospective karyotype analysis in adult acute lymphoblastic leukemia: the cancer and leukemia Group B experience.Blood.**
  Author(s): Wetzler M, Dodge RK, Mrozek K, Carroll AJ, Tantravahi R, Block AW, Pettenati MJ, Le Beau MM, Frankel SR, Stewart CC, Szatrowski TP, Schiffer CA, Larson RA, Bloomfield CD.
  Source: Blood.
  http://www.ncbi.nlm.nih.gov/entrez/query.fcgi?cmd=Retrieve&db=pubmed&dopt=Abstract&list_uids=10339508&query_hl=1

- **Randomized clinical trials in adult acute lymphoblastic leukemia: which is the question?Haematologica.**
  Author(s): Bassan R.
  Source: Haematologica.
  http://www.ncbi.nlm.nih.gov/entrez/query.fcgi?cmd=Retrieve&db=pubmed&dopt=Abstract&list_uids=9573671&query_hl=1

- **Randomized study comparing 4'-epi-doxorubicin (epirubicin) versus doxorubicin as a part of induction treatment in adult acute lymphoblastic leukemia.Am J Hematol.**
  Author(s): Bhutani M, Kumar L, Vora A, Bhardwaj N, Pathak AK, Singh R, Kochupillai V.
  Source: American Journal of Hematology.
  http://www.ncbi.nlm.nih.gov/entrez/query.fcgi?cmd=Retrieve&db=pubmed&dopt=Abstract&list_uids=12447951&query_hl=1

- **Reduced-intensity stem-cell transplantation for adult acute lymphoblastic leukemia: a retrospective study of 33 patients.Bone Marrow Transplant.**
  Author(s): Hamaki T, Kami M, Kanda Y, Yuji K, Inamoto Y, Kishi Y, Nakai K, Nakayama I, Murashige N, Abe Y, Ueda Y, Hino M, Inoue T, Ago H, Hidaka M, Hayashi T, Yamane T, Uoshima N, Miyakoshi S, Taniguchi S.
  Source: Bone Marrow Transplantation.
  http://www.ncbi.nlm.nih.gov/entrez/query.fcgi?cmd=Retrieve&db=pubmed&dopt=Abstract&list_uids=15756282&query_hl=1

- **Reinforced HEAV'D therapy for adult acute lymphoblastic leukemia: improved results and revised prognostic criteria.Hematol Oncol.**
  Author(s): Bassan R, Battista R, Montaldi A, Rambaldi A, D'Emilio A, Viero P, Borleri G, Buelli M, Dini E, Barbui T.
  Source: Hematological Oncology.
  http://www.ncbi.nlm.nih.gov/entrez/query.fcgi?cmd=Retrieve&db=pubmed&dopt=Abstract&list_uids=8144131&query_hl=1

- **Relationship between Daunorubicin dosage delivered during induction therapy and outcome in adult acute lymphoblastic leukemia.Leukemia.**
  Author(s): Todeschini G, Meneghini V, Pizzolo G, Cassibba V, Ambrosetti A, Veneri D, Nadali G, Zanotti R, Tecchio C, Perona G.
  Source: Leukemia : Official Journal of the Leukemia Society of America, Leukemia Research Fund, U.K.
  http://www.ncbi.nlm.nih.gov/entrez/query.fcgi?cmd=Retrieve&db=pubmed&dopt=Abstract&list_uids=8127142&query_hl=1

- **Relationship between minimal residual disease and outcome in adult acute lymphoblastic leukemia.Blood.**
  Author(s): Brisco J, Hughes E, Neoh SH, Sykes PJ, Bradstock K, Enno A, Szer J, McCaul K, Morley AA.
  Source: Blood.
  http://www.ncbi.nlm.nih.gov/entrez/query.fcgi?cmd=Retrieve&db=pu
  bmed&dopt=Abstract&list_uids=8652840&query_hl=1

- **Remission continuation therapy for adult acute lymphoblastic leukemia. Preliminary results with a multidrug treatment protocol.Chemioterapia.**
  Author(s): Rossi G, Verzura P, Marpicati P, Zaniboni A, Ferremi P, Marini G, Marinone G.
  Source: Chemioterapia : International Journal of the Mediterranean Society of Chemotherapy.
  http://www.ncbi.nlm.nih.gov/entrez/query.fcgi?cmd=Retrieve&db=pu
  bmed&dopt=Abstract&list_uids=6597732&query_hl=1

- **Remission maintenance of adult acute lymphoblastic leukemia.Med Pediatr Oncol.**
  Author(s): Armitage JO, Burns CP.
  Source: Medical and Pediatric Oncology.
  http://www.ncbi.nlm.nih.gov/entrez/query.fcgi?cmd=Retrieve&db=pu
  bmed&dopt=Abstract&list_uids=264999&query_hl=1

- **Rescue therapy combining intermediate-dose cytarabine with amsacrine and etoposide in relapsed adult acute lymphoblastic leukemia.Hematol J.**
  Author(s): Reman O, Buzyn A, Lheritier V, Huguet F, Kuentz M, Stamatoullas A, Delannoy A, Fegueux N, Miclea JM, Boiron JM, Vernant JP, Gardin C, Hacini M, Georges M, Fiere D, Thomas X; Groupe d'Etude et de Traitement de la Leucemie Aigue Lymphoblastique de l'Adulte.
  Source: The Hematology Journal : the Official Journal of the European Haematology Association / Eha.
  http://www.ncbi.nlm.nih.gov/entrez/query.fcgi?cmd=Retrieve&db=pu
  bmed&dopt=Abstract&list_uids=15048062&query_hl=1

- **Results of induction therapy with vincristine and prednisone alone in adult acute lymphoblastic leukemia: report of 43 patients and review of the literature.Am J Hematol.**
  Author(s): Hess CE, Zirkle JW.
  Source: American Journal of Hematology.
  http://www.ncbi.nlm.nih.gov/entrez/query.fcgi?cmd=Retrieve&db=pubmed&dopt=Abstract&list_uids=6958203&query_hl=1

- **Risk groups in adult acute lymphoblastic leukemia.Haematol Blood Transfus.**
  Author(s): Hoelzer D, Thiel E, Loffler H, Ganser A, Heimpel H, Buchner T, Urbanitz D, Koch P, Freund M, Diedrich H, et al.
  Source: Haematology and Blood Transfusion.
  http://www.ncbi.nlm.nih.gov/entrez/query.fcgi?cmd=Retrieve&db=pubmed&dopt=Abstract&list_uids=3305188&query_hl=1

- **Risk-adapted treatment of adult acute lymphoblastic leukemia (ALL).Leukemia.**
  Author(s): Linker CA.
  Source: Leukemia : Official Journal of the Leukemia Society of America, Leukemia Research Fund, U.K.
  http://www.ncbi.nlm.nih.gov/entrez/query.fcgi?cmd=Retrieve&db=pubmed&dopt=Abstract&list_uids=9179278&query_hl=1

- **Role of anthracyclines in the treatment of adult acute lymphoblastic leukemia.Acta Haematol.**
  Author(s): Bassan R, Lerede T, Rambaldi A, Barbui T.
  Source: Acta Haematologica.
  http://www.ncbi.nlm.nih.gov/entrez/query.fcgi?cmd=Retrieve&db=pubmed&dopt=Abstract&list_uids=8677741&query_hl=1

- **Role of early anthracycline dose-intensity according to expression of Philadelphia chromosome/BCR-ABL rearrangements in B-precursor adult acute lymphoblastic leukemia.Hematol J.**
  Author(s): Bassan R, Rohatiner AZ, Lerede T, Di Bona E, Rambaldi A, Pogliani E, Rossi G, Fabris P, Morandi S, Casula P, Carter M, Lambertenghi-Deliliers G, Lister TA, Barbui T.
  Source: The Hematology Journal : the Official Journal of the European Haematology Association / Eha.
  http://www.ncbi.nlm.nih.gov/entrez/query.fcgi?cmd=Retrieve&db=pubmed&dopt=Abstract&list_uids=11920195&query_hl=1

- **Role of liposomal daunorubicin, fludarabine and cytarabine (FLAD) in the salvage therapy of adult acute lymphoblastic leukemia.Leuk Lymphoma.**
  Author(s): Clavio M, Pierri I, Venturino C, Garrone A, Canepa L, Miglino M, Varaldo R, Ballerini F, Michelis GL, Balocco M, Abdall N, Gatto S, Gobbi M.
  Source: Leukemia & Lymphoma.
  http://www.ncbi.nlm.nih.gov/entrez/query.fcgi?cmd=Retrieve&db=pubmed&dopt=Abstract&list_uids=15621773&query_hl=1

- **Secondary haematological neoplasm after treatment of adult acute lymphoblastic leukemia: analysis of 1170 adult ALL patients enrolled in the GIMEMA trials. Gruppo Italiano Malattie Ematologiche Maligne dell'Adulto.Br J Haematol.**
  Author(s): Pagano L, Annino L, Ferrari A, Camera A, Martino B, Montillo M, Tosti ME, Mele A, Pulsoni A, Vegna ML, Leone G, Mandelli F.
  Source: British Journal of Haematology.
  http://www.ncbi.nlm.nih.gov/entrez/query.fcgi?cmd=Retrieve&db=pubmed&dopt=Abstract&list_uids=9531332&query_hl=1

- **Sequential induction chemotherapy with vincristine, daunorubicin, cyclophosphamide, and prednisone in adult acute lymphoblastic leukemia.Ann Hematol.**
  Author(s): Thomas X, Danaila C, Bach QK, Dufour P, Christian B, Corront B, Bosly A, Bastion Y, Gratecos N, Leblay R, et al.
  Source: Annals of Hematology.
  http://www.ncbi.nlm.nih.gov/entrez/query.fcgi?cmd=Retrieve&db=pubmed&dopt=Abstract&list_uids=7880925&query_hl=1

- **Short-term intensive treatment (V.A.A.P.) of adult acute lymphoblastic leukemia and lymphoblastic lymphoma.Eur J Haematol.**
  Author(s): Willemze R, Peters WG, Colly LP.
  Source: European Journal of Haematology.
  http://www.ncbi.nlm.nih.gov/entrez/query.fcgi?cmd=Retrieve&db=pubmed&dopt=Abstract&list_uids=3208871&query_hl=1

- **Successful treatment of adult acute lymphoblastic leukemia after relapse with prednisone, intermediate-dose cytarabine, mitoxantrone, and etoposide (PAME) chemotherapy.Cancer.**
  Author(s): Milpied N, Gisselbrecht C, Harousseau JL, Sebban C, Witz F, Troussard X, Gratecos N, Michallet M, LeBlond V, Auzanneau G, et al.
  Source: Cancer.
  http://www.ncbi.nlm.nih.gov/entrez/query.fcgi?cmd=Retrieve&db=pubmed&dopt=Abstract&list_uids=2386891&query_hl=1

- **Susceptibility of adult acute lymphoblastic leukemia blasts to lysis by lymphokine-activated killer cells.Leukemia.**
  Author(s): Archimbaud E, Thomas X, Campos L, Magaud JP, Fiere D, Dore JF.
  Source: Leukemia : Official Journal of the Leukemia Society of America, Leukemia Research Fund, U.K.
  http://www.ncbi.nlm.nih.gov/entrez/query.fcgi?cmd=Retrieve&db=pubmed&dopt=Abstract&list_uids=1961038&query_hl=1

- **Systemic high-dose ara-C for the treatment of meningeal leukemia in adult acute lymphoblastic leukemia and non-Hodgkin's lymphoma.J Clin Oncol.**
  Author(s): Morra E, Lazzarino M, Inverardi D, Brusamolino E, Orlandi E, Canevari A, Pagnucco G, Bernasconi C.
  Source: Journal of Clinical Oncology : Official Journal of the American Society of Clinical Oncology.
  http://www.ncbi.nlm.nih.gov/entrez/query.fcgi?cmd=Retrieve&db=pubmed&dopt=Abstract&list_uids=3461134&query_hl=1

- **TdT in adult acute lymphoblastic leukemia: relationship with blast cell count.Haematologica.**
  Author(s): Baccarani M, Marini M, Bagnara GP, Gobbi M, Saviotti F, Brunelli MA, Tura S.
  Source: Haematologica.
  http://www.ncbi.nlm.nih.gov/entrez/query.fcgi?cmd=Retrieve&db=pubmed&dopt=Abstract&list_uids=6796467&query_hl=1

- **TEL/AML1 fusion gene is a rare event in adult acute lymphoblastic leukemia.Leukemia.**
  Author(s): Raynaud S, Mauvieux L, Cayuela JM, Bastard C, Bilhou-Nabera C, Debuire B, Bories D, Boucheix C, Charrin C, Fiere D, Gabert J.
  Source: Leukemia : Official Journal of the Leukemia Society of America, Leukemia Research Fund, U.K.
  http://www.ncbi.nlm.nih.gov/entrez/query.fcgi?cmd=Retrieve&db=pubmed&dopt=Abstract&list_uids=8751475&query_hl=1

- **Teniposide (VM-26) and ara-C in the treatment of adult acute lymphoblastic leukemia.Semin Oncol.**
  Author(s): Linker CA, Levitt LJ, O'Donnell M, Ries CA, Forman SJ.
  Source: Seminars in Oncology.
  http://www.ncbi.nlm.nih.gov/entrez/query.fcgi?cmd=Retrieve&db=pubmed&dopt=Abstract&list_uids=3473686&query_hl=1

- **Teniposide and cytarabine combination chemotherapy in the treatment of relapsed adolescent and adult acute lymphoblastic leukemia.Cancer Treat Rep.**
  Author(s): Sanz GF, Sanz MA, Rafecas FJ, Martinez JA, Martin-Aragones G, Marty ML.
  Source: Cancer Treatment Reports.
  http://www.ncbi.nlm.nih.gov/entrez/query.fcgi?cmd=Retrieve&db=pubmed&dopt=Abstract&list_uids=3464352&query_hl=1

- **The aplastic presentation of adult acute lymphoblastic leukemia.Br J Haematol.**
  Author(s): Nakamori Y, Takahashi M, Moriyama Y, Httori A, Shibata A, Watanabe T, Oda Y.
  Source: British Journal of Haematology.
  http://www.ncbi.nlm.nih.gov/entrez/query.fcgi?cmd=Retrieve&db=pubmed&dopt=Abstract&list_uids=3457602&query_hl=1

- **The biology and therapy of adult acute lymphoblastic leukemia.Cancer.**
  Author(s): Faderl S, Jeha S, Kantarjian HM.
  Source: Cancer.
  http://www.ncbi.nlm.nih.gov/entrez/query.fcgi?cmd=Retrieve&db=pubmed&dopt=Abstract&list_uids=14508819&query_hl=1

- **The expression of the multidrug resistance related glycoprotein in adult acute lymphoblastic leukemia.Haematologica.**
  Author(s): Savignano C, Geromin A, Michieli M, Damiani D, Michelutti A, Melli C, Fanin R, Baccarani M.
  Source: Haematologica.
  http://www.ncbi.nlm.nih.gov/entrez/query.fcgi?cmd=Retrieve&db=pubmed&dopt=Abstract&list_uids=7906239&query_hl=1

- **The prognostic significance of p16INK4a/p14ARF and p15INK4b deletions in adult acute lymphoblastic leukemia.Clin Cancer Res.**
  Author(s): Faderl S, Kantarjian HM, Manshouri T, Chan CY, Pierce S, Hays KJ, Cortes J, Thomas D, Estrov Z, Albitar M.
  Source: Clinical Cancer Research : an Official Journal of the American Association for Cancer Research.
  http://www.ncbi.nlm.nih.gov/entrez/query.fcgi?cmd=Retrieve&db=pubmed&dopt=Abstract&list_uids=10430092&query_hl=1

- **The role of posttransplantation maintenance chemotherapy in improving the outcome of autotransplantation in adult acute lymphoblastic leukemia.Blood.**
  Author(s): Powles R, Sirohi B, Treleaven J, Kulkarni S, Tait D, Singhal S, Mehta J.
  Source: Blood.
  http://www.ncbi.nlm.nih.gov/entrez/query.fcgi?cmd=Retrieve&db=pubmed&dopt=Abstract&list_uids=12176883&query_hl=1

- **The U.S. trials in adult acute lymphoblastic leukemia.Ann Hematol.**
  Author(s): Larson RA.
  Source: Annals of Hematology.
  http://www.ncbi.nlm.nih.gov/entrez/query.fcgi?cmd=Retrieve&db=pubmed&dopt=Abstract&list_uids=15124704&query_hl=1

- **The use of anthracyclines in adult acute lymphoblastic leukemia.Haematologica.**
  Author(s): Bassan R, Lerede T, Rambaldi A, Buelli M, Viero P, Barbui T.
  Source: Haematologica.
  http://www.ncbi.nlm.nih.gov/entrez/query.fcgi?cmd=Retrieve&db=pubmed&dopt=Abstract&list_uids=7672723&query_hl=1

- **The value of high-dose systemic chemotherapy and intrathecal therapy for central nervous system prophylaxis in different risk groups of adult acute lymphoblastic leukemia.Blood.**
  Author(s): Cortes J, O'Brien SM, Pierce S, Keating MJ, Freireich EJ, Kantarjian HM.
  Source: Blood.
  http://www.ncbi.nlm.nih.gov/entrez/query.fcgi?cmd=Retrieve&db=pubmed&dopt=Abstract&list_uids=7662956&query_hl=1

- **Therapy for adolescent and adult acute lymphoblastic leukemia: randomization of induction and consolidation therapies (preliminary results of EORTC Study 58791).Haematol Blood Transfus.**
  Author(s): Stryckmans P, Marie JP, Suciu S, Solbu G, Debusscher L, Bury J, Peetermans M, Andrien JM, Fiere D, Cauchie C, et al.
  Source: Haematology and Blood Transfusion.
  http://www.ncbi.nlm.nih.gov/entrez/query.fcgi?cmd=Retrieve&db=pubmed&dopt=Abstract&list_uids=3305190&query_hl=1

- **Therapy of refractory adult acute lymphoblastic leukemia with vincristine and prednisone plus tandem methotrexate and L-asparaginase. Results of a Cancer and Leukemia Group B Study.Am J Clin Oncol.**
  Author(s): Terebelo HR, Anderson K, Wiernik PH, Cuttner J, Cooper RM, Faso L, Berenberg JL.
  Source: American Journal of Clinical Oncology : the Official Publication of the American Radium Society.
  http://www.ncbi.nlm.nih.gov/entrez/query.fcgi?cmd=Retrieve&db=pubmed&dopt=Abstract&list_uids=3465228&query_hl=1

- **Therapy-related adult acute lymphoblastic leukemia with t(4;11)(q21; q23): MLL rearrangement, p53 mutation and multilineage involvement.Leukemia.**
  Author(s): Bigoni R, Cuneo A, Roberti MG, Moretti S, De Angeli C, Dabusti M, Campioni D, del Senno L, Biondi A, Chaplin T, Young BD, Castoldi G.
  Source: Leukemia : Official Journal of the Leukemia Society of America, Leukemia Research Fund, U.K.
  http://www.ncbi.nlm.nih.gov/entrez/query.fcgi?cmd=Retrieve&db=pubmed&dopt=Abstract&list_uids=10374873&query_hl=1

- **Thrombosis associated with L-asparaginase therapy and low fibrinogen levels in adult acute lymphoblastic leukemia.Am J Hematol.**
  Author(s): Beinart G, Damon L.
  Source: American Journal of Hematology.
  http://www.ncbi.nlm.nih.gov/entrez/query.fcgi?cmd=Retrieve&db=pu
  bmed&dopt=Abstract&list_uids=15551293&query_hl=1

- **Towards an integrated classification of adult acute lymphoblastic leukemia.Rev Clin Exp Hematol.**
  Author(s): Foa R, Vitale A.
  Source: Reviews in Clinical and Experimental Hematology.
  http://www.ncbi.nlm.nih.gov/entrez/query.fcgi?cmd=Retrieve&db=pu
  bmed&dopt=Abstract&list_uids=12196215&query_hl=1

- **Transient aplasia preceding adult acute lymphoblastic leukemia.Haematologica.**
  Author(s): D'Alessio A, Invernizzi R, Bernuzzi S, Fiamenghi C, Giusto M, Iannone AM.
  Source: Haematologica.
  http://www.ncbi.nlm.nih.gov/entrez/query.fcgi?cmd=Retrieve&db=pu
  bmed&dopt=Abstract&list_uids=8349189&query_hl=1

- **Translocation t(8;14)(q24;q32) and del(1)(p22) in FAB-L1 adult acute lymphoblastic leukemia with long survival.Cancer Genet Cytogenet.**
  Author(s): Carbone P, Barbata G, Tumminello P, Bellanca F, Majolino I, Granata G.
  Source: Cancer Genetics and Cytogenetics.
  http://www.ncbi.nlm.nih.gov/entrez/query.fcgi?cmd=Retrieve&db=pu
  bmed&dopt=Abstract&list_uids=3162704&query_hl=1

- **Treatment of adult acute lymphoblastic leukemia (ALL): long-term follow-up of the GIMEMA ALL 0288 randomized study.Blood.**
  Author(s): Annino L, Vegna ML, Camera A, Specchia G, Visani G, Fioritoni G, Ferrara F, Peta A, Ciolli S, Deplano W, Fabbiano F, Sica S, Di Raimondo F, Cascavilla N, Tabilio A, Leoni P, Invernizzi R, Baccarani M, Rotoli B, Amadori S, Mandelli F; GIMEMA Group.
  Source: Blood.
  http://www.ncbi.nlm.nih.gov/entrez/query.fcgi?cmd=Retrieve&db=pu
  bmed&dopt=Abstract&list_uids=11806988&query_hl=1

- **Treatment of adult acute lymphoblastic leukemia with adriamycin, vincristine, and prednisone.Med Pediatr Oncol.**
  Author(s): Aviles A, Sinco A, Rivera R, Ambriz R, Herrera JG, Pizzuto J.
  Source: Medical and Pediatric Oncology.
  http://www.ncbi.nlm.nih.gov/entrez/query.fcgi?cmd=Retrieve&db=pu
  bmed&dopt=Abstract&list_uids=6572781&query_hl=1

- **Treatment of adult acute lymphoblastic leukemia with allogeneic bone marrow transplantation. Multivariate analysis of factors affecting acute graft-versus-host disease, relapse, and relapse-free survival.Bone Marrow Transplant.**
  Author(s): Doney K, Fisher LD, Appelbaum FR, Buckner CD, Storb R, Singer J, Fefer A, Anasetti C, Beatty P, Bensinger W, et al.
  Source: Bone Marrow Transplantation.
  http://www.ncbi.nlm.nih.gov/entrez/query.fcgi?cmd=Retrieve&db=pu
  bmed&dopt=Abstract&list_uids=1873592&query_hl=1

- **Treatment of adult acute lymphoblastic leukemia with cytosine arabinoside, vincristine, and prednisone.Cancer Treat Rep.**
  Author(s): Gingrich RD, Armitage JO, Burns CP.
  Source: Cancer Treatment Reports.
  http://www.ncbi.nlm.nih.gov/entrez/query.fcgi?cmd=Retrieve&db=pu
  bmed&dopt=Abstract&list_uids=356988&query_hl=1

- **Treatment of adult acute lymphoblastic leukemia with intensive cyclical chemotherapy: a follow-up report.Blood.**
  Author(s): Linker CA, Levitt LJ, O'Donnell M, Forman SJ, Ries CA.
  Source: Blood.
  http://www.ncbi.nlm.nih.gov/entrez/query.fcgi?cmd=Retrieve&db=pu
  bmed&dopt=Abstract&list_uids=1835410&query_hl=1

- **Treatment of adult acute lymphoblastic leukemia. Preliminary results of a trial from the French Group.Haematol Blood Transfus.**
  Author(s): Fiere D, Archimbaud E, Extra JM, Marty M, David B, Witz F, Sotto JJ, Rochant H, Gastaut JA, Le Prise PY.
  Source: Haematology and Blood Transfusion.
  http://www.ncbi.nlm.nih.gov/entrez/query.fcgi?cmd=Retrieve&db=pu
  bmed&dopt=Abstract&list_uids=3305189&query_hl=1

- **Treatment of adult acute lymphoblastic leukemia.Semin Oncol.**
  Author(s): Laport GF, Larson RA.
  Source: Seminars in Oncology.
  http://www.ncbi.nlm.nih.gov/entrez/query.fcgi?cmd=Retrieve&db=pu
  bmed&dopt=Abstract&list_uids=9045306&query_hl=1

- **Treatment of adult acute lymphoblastic leukemia: results of two trials.Neoplasma.**
  Author(s): Koza I, Cerny V, Horak I, Bohunicky L, Gyarfas J, Svancarova L, Hal'ko J, Mardiak J, Zonnenschein T, Thalmeinerova Z.
  Source: Neoplasma.
  http://www.ncbi.nlm.nih.gov/entrez/query.fcgi?cmd=Retrieve&db=pu
  bmed&dopt=Abstract&list_uids=7027059&query_hl=1

- **Treatment of relapsed adult acute lymphoblastic leukemia with fludarabine and cytosine arabinoside followed by granulocyte colony-stimulating factor (FLAG-GCSF).Leuk Lymphoma.**
  Author(s): Montillo M, Tedeschi A, Centurioni R, Leoni P.
  Source: Leukemia & Lymphoma.
  http://www.ncbi.nlm.nih.gov/entrez/query.fcgi?cmd=Retrieve&db=pu
  bmed&dopt=Abstract&list_uids=9250830&query_hl=1

- **Treatment options for newly diagnosed patients with adult acute lymphoblastic leukemia.Curr Hematol Rep.**
  Author(s): Lamanna N, Weiss M.
  Source: Current Hematology Reports.
  http://www.ncbi.nlm.nih.gov/entrez/query.fcgi?cmd=Retrieve&db=pu
  bmed&dopt=Abstract&list_uids=14695849&query_hl=1

- **Tumor suppressor gene alteration in adult acute lymphoblastic leukemia (ALL). Analysis of retinoblastoma (Rb) and p53 gene expression in lymphoblasts of patients with de novo, relapsed, or refractory ALL treated in Southwest Oncology Group studies.Leukemia.**
  Author(s): Tsai T, Davalath S, Rankin C, Radich JP, Head D, Appelbaum FR, Boldt DH.
  Source: Leukemia : Official Journal of the Leukemia Society of America, Leukemia Research Fund, U.K.
  http://www.ncbi.nlm.nih.gov/entrez/query.fcgi?cmd=Retrieve&db=pu
  bmed&dopt=Abstract&list_uids=8946929&query_hl=1

- **Ultrastructural cytochemical prospective study of adult acute lymphoblastic leukemia: detection of peroxidase activity in patients failing to respond to treatment.Cancer.**
  Author(s): Reiffers J, Darmendrail V, Larrue J, Villenave I, Bernard P, Boisseau M, Broustet A.
  Source: Cancer.
  http://www.ncbi.nlm.nih.gov/entrez/query.fcgi?cmd=Retrieve&db=pubmed&dopt=Abstract&list_uids=6944143&query_hl=1

- **Use of prognostic factors in deciding therapy for adult acute lymphoblastic leukemia: new approaches at Memorial Sloan-Kettering Cancer Center (MSKCC).Bone Marrow Transplant.**
  Author(s): Gulati SC, Gaynor J, Esseesse I, Gee T, Little C, Andreeff M, Berman E, Kempin S, Clarkson B.
  Source: Bone Marrow Transplantation.
  http://www.ncbi.nlm.nih.gov/entrez/query.fcgi?cmd=Retrieve&db=pubmed&dopt=Abstract&list_uids=2653525&query_hl=1

- **Value of immunophenotype in intensively treated adult acute lymphoblastic leukemia: cancer and leukemia Group B study 8364.Blood.**
  Author(s): Czuczman MS, Dodge RK, Stewart CC, Frankel SR, Davey FR, Powell BL, Szatrowski TP, Schiffer CA, Larson RA, Bloomfield CD.
  Source: Blood.
  http://www.ncbi.nlm.nih.gov/entrez/query.fcgi?cmd=Retrieve&db=pubmed&dopt=Abstract&list_uids=10339502&query_hl=1

- **VLA-4 and VLA-5 integrin expression in adult acute lymphoblastic leukemia.Exp Hematol.**
  Author(s): Stagno F, Cacciola E, Guglielmo P, Cacciola RR, Cacciola E.
  Source: Experimental Hematology.
  http://www.ncbi.nlm.nih.gov/entrez/query.fcgi?cmd=Retrieve&db=pubmed&dopt=Abstract&list_uids=8608797&query_hl=1

- **VM-26 and cytarabine combination chemotherapy in refractory or relapsed adult acute lymphoblastic leukemia.Haematologica.**
  Author(s): Carella AM, Santini G, Martinengo M, Giordano D, Nati S, Congiu A, Risso M, Vimercati R, Cerri R, Rossi E, et al.
  Source: Haematologica.
  http://www.ncbi.nlm.nih.gov/entrez/query.fcgi?cmd=Retrieve&db=pubmed&dopt=Abstract&list_uids=6441752&query_hl=1

Vocabulary Builder

The following vocabulary builder provides definitions of words used in this chapter that have not been defined in previous chapters:

CDNA: Synthetic DNA reverse transcribed from a specific RNA through the action of the enzyme reverse transcriptase. DNA synthesized by reverse transcriptase using RNA as a template. [NIH]

Cofactor: A substance, microorganism or environmental factor that activates or enhances the action of another entity such as a disease-causing agent. [NIH]

Consolidation: The healing process of a bone fracture. [NIH]

Deletion: A genetic rearrangement through loss of segments of DNA (chromosomes), bringing sequences, which are normally separated, into close proximity. [NIH]

Haematology: The science of the blood, its nature, functions, and diseases. [NIH]

Immunologic: The ability of the antibody-forming system to recall a previous experience with an antigen and to respond to a second exposure with the prompt production of large amounts of antibody. [NIH]

Karyotype: The characteristic chromosome complement of an individual, race, or species as defined by their number, size, shape, etc. [NIH]

Lymphokine: A soluble protein produced by some types of white blood cell that stimulates other white blood cells to kill foreign invaders. [NIH]

Monoclonal: An antibody produced by culturing a single type of cell. It therefore consists of a single species of immunoglobulin molecules. [NIH]

Morphological: Relating to the configuration or the structure of live organs. [NIH]

MRNA: The RNA molecule that conveys from the DNA the information that is to be translated into the structure of a particular polypeptide molecule. [NIH]

Pharmacodynamic: Is concerned with the response of living tissues to chemical stimuli, that is, the action of drugs on the living organism in the absence of disease. [NIH]

Phenotypes: An organism as observed, i. e. as judged by its visually perceptible characters resulting from the interaction of its genotype with the environment. [NIH]

Polymerase: An enzyme which catalyses the synthesis of DNA using a single DNA strand as a template. The polymerase copies the template in the 5'-3'direction provided that sufficient quantities of free nucleotides, dATP and dTTP are present. [NIH]

Probe: An instrument used in exploring cavities, or in the detection and dilatation of strictures, or in demonstrating the potency of channels; an elongated instrument for exploring or sounding body cavities. [NIH]

Protocol: The detailed plan for a clinical trial that states the trial's rationale, purpose, drug or vaccine dosages, length of study, routes of administration, who may participate, and other aspects of trial design. [NIH]

Rankin: A three-bladed clamp. [NIH]

Recombination: The formation of new combinations of genes as a result of segregation in crosses between genetically different parents; also the rearrangement of linked genes due to crossing-over. [NIH]

Reductase: Enzyme converting testosterone to dihydrotestosterone. [NIH]

Suppression: A conscious exclusion of disapproved desire contrary with repression, in which the process of exclusion is not conscious. [NIH]

Translocation: The movement of material in solution inside the body of the plant. [NIH]

Triad: Trivalent. [NIH]

Vitro: Descriptive of an event or enzyme reaction under experimental investigation occurring outside a living organism. Parts of an organism or microorganism are used together with artificial substrates and/or conditions. [NIH]

Zoster: A virus infection of the Gasserian ganglion and its nerve branches, characterized by discrete areas of vesiculation of the epithelium of the forehead, the nose, the eyelids, and the cornea together with subepithelial infiltration. [NIH]

Chapter 4. Patents on Adult Acute Lymphoblastic Leukemia

Overview

You can learn about innovations relating to adult acute lymphoblastic leukemia by reading recent patents and patent applications. Patents can be physical innovations (e.g. chemicals, pharmaceuticals, medical equipment) or processes (e.g. treatments or diagnostic procedures). The United States Patent and Trademark Office defines a patent as a grant of a property right to the inventor, issued by the Patent and Trademark Office.[21] Patents, therefore, are intellectual property. For the United States, the term of a new patent is 20 years from the date when the patent application was filed. If the inventor wishes to receive economic benefits, it is likely that the invention will become commercially available to patients with adult acute lymphoblastic leukemia within 20 years of the initial filing. It is important to understand, therefore, that an inventor's patent does not indicate that a product or service is or will be commercially available to patients with adult acute lymphoblastic leukemia. The patent implies only that the inventor has "the right to exclude others from making, using, offering for sale, or selling" the invention in the United States. While this relates to U.S. patents, similar rules govern foreign patents.

In this chapter, we show you how to locate information on patents and their inventors. If you find a patent that is particularly interesting to you, contact the inventor or the assignee for further information.

---

[21]Adapted from The U. S. Patent and Trademark Office:
http://www.uspto.gov/web/offices/pac/doc/general/whatis.htm.

Patents on Adult Acute Lymphoblastic Leukemia

By performing a patent search focusing on adult acute lymphoblastic leukemia, you can obtain information such as the title of the invention, the names of the inventor(s), the assignee(s) or the company that owns or controls the patent, a short abstract that summarizes the patent, and a few excerpts from the description of the patent. The abstract of a patent tends to be more technical in nature, while the description is often written for the public. Full patent descriptions contain much more information than is presented here (e.g. claims, references, figures, diagrams, etc.). We will tell you how to obtain this information later in the chapter. The following is an example of the type of information that you can expect to obtain from a patent search on adult acute lymphoblastic leukemia:

- **BRC/ABL transgenic animals as models for Philadelphia chromosome positive chronic myelogenous and acute lymphoblastic leukemia**

  Inventor(s): Groffen; John (Los Angeles, CA), Heisterkamp; Nora (Los Angeles, CA), Pattengale; Paul K. (Los Angeles, CA)

  Assignee(s): Childrens Hospital of Los Angeles (Los Angeles, CA)

  Patent Number: 5,491,283

  Date filed: January 14, 1993

  Abstract: The present invention relates to non-human transgenic animals which contain a transgene comprising a BCR/ABL gene fusion and which develop leukemia. In a preferred embodiment of the present invention, the transgenic animals exhibit a rapid induction of acute leukemia.The present invention offers the advantage of providing, for the first time, a non-human transgenic animal model system which carries the BCR/ABL gene fusion characteristic of the Philadelphia chromosome and which develops leukemia in a manner directly analogous to the clinical progression of chronic myelogenous leukemia (CML) and/or **acute lymphoblastic leukemia** (ALL) in humans. This model system for human leukemia may be valuable in obtaining a better understanding of CML and ALL and in developing effective therapeutic regimens.

  Excerpt(s): The present invention relates to transgenic non-human animals which contain a transgene comprising a BCR/ABL gene fusion and which develop leukemia. The nonhuman transgenic animals of the invention may serve as valuable models for chronic myelogenous and **acute lymphoblastic leukemia** in humans... Leukemia is a malignant condition of white blood cells in which bone marrow is diffusely replaced by relatively immature white blood cells which generally also appear, in large numbers, in the circulating blood (Robbins and Angell, 1976, in "Basic Pathology", Second Edition, W. B. Saunders Co., Philadelphia, pp. 349-354). Leukemias may be classified as acute lymphocytic (or lymphoblastic), chronic lymphocytic, acute myelogenous, or chronic myelogenous... Chronic myelogenous leukemia (CML) accounts for approximately 25 percent of all leukemias. Onset of the disease occurs most frequently in middle age, with males and females affected approximately equally. CML is generally associated with prominent enlargement of the spleen. Prognosis for survival is approximately three to four years.

Web site: http://www.delphion.com/details?pn=US05491283__

- **Process for preparation of a biomarker specific for O-acetylated sialic acid useful for diagnosing, monitoring treatment outcome, and predicting relapse of lymphoblastic leukemia**

Inventor(s): Chatterjee; Mitali (Indian Institute of Chemical Biology, 4 Raja S.C. Mullick Road, Jadavpur, Calcutta, IN 700 032), Mandal; Chitra (Indian Institute of Chemical Biology, 4 Raja S.C. Mullick Road, Jadavpur, Calcutta, IN 700 032), Pal; Santanu (Indian Institute of Chemical Biology, 4 Raja S.C. Mullick Road, Jadavpur, Calcutta, IN 700 032)

Assignee(s): none reported

Patent Number: 6,693,177

Date filed: December 3, 1999

Abstract: The invention relates to a novel process for preparation of a biomarker specific for O-acetylated sialic acid and useful for the diagnosis, monitoring outcome of treatment and prediction of relapse of **acute lymphoblastic leukemia,** said process comprising the steps of (I) separating serum from the blood of patients of **acute lymphoblastic leukemia;** (ii) separation of low molecular weight fractions and galactose binding proteins from the serum on affinity matrix; (iii) passing the galactose free protein fraction obtained in step (ii) over another affinity matrix to capture O-acetyl sialic acid specific protein fraction; (iv) eluting specific protein fraction with a buffer at alkaline pH in the range of 8.0-11.0 followed by immediate neutralization of the fraction; (v) passing O-acetyl sialic acid specific protein obtained in step (iv) over Agarose column to get O-acetyl sialic acid specific antibody and eluting the said antibody with an appropriate buffer at acidic pH, followed by immediate neutralization of the fraction and dialyzing the neutralized protein to get purified disease specific antibody as biomarker and a method of diagnosing, monitoring outcome of treatment and prediction of relapse of

acute lymphoblastic leukemia using the biomarker obtained by the novel process.

Excerpt(s): The present invention relates to a novel process for the preparation of a biomarker which is an antibody for O-acetylated sialic acid and useful for the diagnosis, monitoring outcome of treatment and prediction of relapse of **acute lymphoblastic leukemia.** More particularly, the present invention relates to a novel process for the preparation of O-acetylated sialic protein immunoglobin useful as a biomarker for the diagnosis of **acute lymphoblastic leukemia.** Leukemia is a heterogeneous group of neoplastic cells arising from the malignant transformation of hematopoietic (i.e. blood forming) cells. Leukemia can be broadly classified according to the cell type involved myeloid or lymphoid and as acute and chronic depending on the natural history of the disease. **Acute lymphoblastic leukemia** (ALL) is the commonest type of leukemnia in children and adolescents. It occurs in all races with a peak incidence in children between 3 and 5 years of age. ALL is diagnosed in 2000-3000 new cases of children in the United States every year, whereas acute myelogenous leukemia is diagnosed in only 500 children and chronic myeloid leukemia in fewer than 100. About 40 million children under the age group of 15 years are affected and nearly about 75% of these have ALL. Pediatric hematopoietic malignancies rank first in cancer incidence and mortality in children and are responsible for roughly 40% of childhood related death... The causes of leukemia are not known but environmental agents including irradiation, chemical carcinogens, cytogenetic abnormalities and retrovirus infections are known to play an important role in the etiology of leukemia. For instance, individual with occupational radiation exposure, patients receiving radiation therapy or Japanese survivors of the atomic bomb explosions have a predictable and dose related increased incidence of leukemia.

Web site: http://www.delphion.com/details?pn=US06693177__

Keeping Current

In order to stay informed about patents and patent applications dealing with adult acute lymphoblastic leukemia, you can access the U.S. Patent Office archive via the Internet at the following Web address: **http://www.uspto.gov/patft/index.html**. You will see two broad options: (1) Issued Patent, and (2) Published Applications. To see a list of issued patents, perform the following steps: Under "Issued Patents," click "Quick Search." Then, type "adult acute lymphoblastic leukemia" (or synonyms) into the "Term 1" box. After clicking on the search button, scroll down to see the various patents which have been granted to date on adult acute lymphoblastic leukemia.

You can also use this procedure to view pending patent applications concerning adult acute lymphoblastic leukemia. Simply go back to the following Web address: **http://www.uspto.gov/patft/index.html**. Select "Quick Search" under "Published Applications." Then proceed with the steps listed above.

CHAPTER 5. PHYSICIAN GUIDELINES AND DATABASES

Overview

Doctors and medical researchers rely on a number of information sources to help patients with their conditions. Many will subscribe to journals or newsletters published by their professional associations or refer to specialized textbooks or clinical guides published for the medical profession. In this chapter, we focus on databases and Internet-based guidelines created or written for this professional audience.

NIH Guidelines

For the more common diseases, The National Institutes of Health publish guidelines that are frequently consulted by physicians. Publications are typically written by one or more of the various NIH Institutes. For physician guidelines, commonly referred to as "clinical" or "professional" guidelines, you can visit the following Institutes:

- Office of the Director (OD); guidelines consolidated across agencies available at **http://www.nih.gov/health/consumer/conkey.htm**

- National Institute of General Medical Sciences (NIGMS); fact sheets available at **http://www.nigms.nih.gov/news/facts/**

- National Library of Medicine (NLM); extensive encyclopedia (A.D.A.M., Inc.) with guidelines:
  http://www.nlm.nih.gov/medlineplus/healthtopics.html

- National Cancer Institute (NCI); guidelines available at
  http://www.cancer.gov/cancerinfo/list.aspx?viewid=5f35036e-5497-4d86-8c2c-714a9f7c8d25

In this chapter, we begin by reproducing one such guideline for adult acute lymphoblastic leukemia:

What Is Adult Acute Lymphoblastic Leukemia?[22]

Sixty percent to 80% of adults with acute lymphoblastic leukemia (ALL) can be expected to attain complete remission status following appropriate induction therapy. Approximately 35% to 40% of adults with ALL can be expected to survive 2 years with aggressive induction combination chemotherapy and effective supportive care during induction therapy (appropriate early treatment of infection, hyperuricemia, and bleeding). A few studies that use intensive multiagent approaches suggest that a 50% 3-year survival is achievable in selected patients, but these results must be verified by other investigators.[23]

As in childhood ALL, adult patients with ALL are at risk of developing central nervous system (CNS) involvement during the course of their disease. This is particularly true for patients with L3 histology.[24] Both treatment and prognosis are influenced by this complication. The examination of bone marrow aspirates and/or biopsy specimens should be done by an experienced oncologist, hematologist, hematopathologist, or general pathologist who is capable of interpreting conventional and specially stained specimens. Diagnostic confusion with acute myelocytic leukemia (AML), hairy-cell leukemia, and malignant lymphoma is not uncommon. Proper diagnosis is crucial because of the difference in prognosis and treatment of ALL and AML. Immunophenotypic analysis is essential because

---

[22] The following guidelines appeared on the NCI Web site on February 9, 2004. The text was last modified in October 2003. The text has been adapted for this sourcebook.

[23] Gaynor J, Chapman D, Little C, et al.: A cause-specific hazard rate analysis of prognostic factors among 199 adults with acute lymphoblastic leukemia: the Memorial Hospital experience since 1969. Journal of Clinical Oncology 6(6): 1014-1030, 1988.

Hoelzer D, Thiel E, Loffler H, et al.: Prognostic factors in a multicenter study for treatment of acute lymphoblastic leukemia in adults. Blood 71(1): 123-131, 1988.

Zhang MJ, Hoelzer D, Horowitz MM, et al.: Long-term follow-up of adults with acute lymphoblastic leukemia in first remission treated with chemotherapy or bone marrow transplantation. Annals of Internal Medicine 123(6): 428-431, 1995.

Larson RA, Dodge RK, Burns CP, et al.: A five-drug remission induction regimen with intensive consolidation for adults with acute lymphoblastic leukemia: Cancer and Leukemia Group B study 8811. Blood 85(8): 2025-2037, 1995.

[24] Kantarjian HM, Walters RS, Smith TL, et al.: Identification of risk groups for development of central nervous system leukemia in adults with acute lymphocytic leukemia. Blood 72(5): 1784-1789, 1988.

leukemias that do not express myeloperoxidase include M0 and M7 AML as well as ALL.

Appropriate initial treatment, usually consisting of a regimen that includes the combination of vincristine, prednisone, and anthracycline, with or without asparaginase, results in a complete remission rate of up to 80%. Median remission duration for the complete responders is approximately 15 months. Entry into a clinical trial is highly desirable to assure adequate patient treatment and also maximal information retrieval from the treatment of this highly responsive, but usually fatal, disease. Patients who experience a relapse after remission can be expected to succumb within 1 year, even if a second complete remission is achieved. If there are appropriate available donors and if the patient is younger than 55 years of age, bone marrow transplantation may be a consideration in the management of this disease.[25] Transplant centers performing 5 or fewer transplants annually usually have poorer results than larger centers.[26] If allogeneic transplant is considered, transfusions with blood products from a potential donor should be avoided if possible.[27]

Age, which is a significant factor in childhood ALL and in AML, may also be an important prognostic factor in adult ALL. In one study, overall the prognosis was better in patients younger than 25 years; another study found a better prognosis in those younger than 35 years. These findings may, in

---

[25] Bortin MM, Horowitz MM, Gale RP, et al.: Changing trends in allogeneic bone marrow transplantation for leukemia in the 1980s. JAMA: Journal of the American Medical Association 268(5): 607-612, 1992.

[26] Horowitz MM, Przepiorka D, Champlin RE, et al.: Should HLA-identical sibling bone marrow transplants for leukemia be restricted to large centers? Blood 79(10): 2771-2774, 1992.

[27] Larson RA, Dodge RK, Burns CP, et al.: A five-drug remission induction regimen with intensive consolidation for adults with acute lymphoblastic leukemia: Cancer and Leukemia Group B study 8811. Blood 85(8): 2025-2037, 1995.

Linker CA, Levitt LJ, O'Donnell M, et al.: Treatment of adult acute lymphoblastic leukemia with intensive cyclical chemotherapy: a follow-up report. Blood 78(11): 2814-2822, 1991.

Barrett AJ, Horowitz MM, Gale RP, et al.: Marrow transplantation for acute lymphoblastic leukemia: factors affecting relapse and survival. Blood 74(2): 862-871, 1989.

Dinsmore R, Kirkpatrick D, Flomenberg N, et al.: Allogeneic bone marrow transplantation for patients with acute lymphoblastic leukemia. Blood 62(2): 381-388, 1983.

Jacobs AD, Gale RP: Recent advances in the biology and treatment of acute lymphoblastic leukemia in adults. New England Journal of Medicine 311(19): 1219-1231, 1984.

Doney K, Buckner CD, Kopecky KJ, et al.: Marrow transplantation for patients with acute lymphoblastic leukemia in first marrow remission. Bone Marrow Transplantation 2(4): 355-363, 1987.

Vernant JP, Marit G, Maraninchi D, et al.: Allogeneic bone marrow transplantation in adults with acute lymphoblastic leukemia in first complete remission. Journal of Clinical Oncology 6(2): 227-231, 1988.

part, be related to the increased incidence of the Philadelphia (Ph) chromosome in older ALL patients, a subgroup associated with poor prognosis.[28] Elevated B2-microglobulin is associated with a poor prognosis in adults as evidenced by lower response rate, increased incidence of CNS involvement, and significantly worse survival.[29] Patients with Ph chromosome-positive ALL are rarely cured with chemotherapy. Many patients who have molecular evidence of the bcr-abl fusion gene, which characterizes the Ph chromosome, have no evidence of the abnormal chromosome by cytogenetics. Because many patients have a different fusion protein from the one found in chronic myelogenous leukemia (p190 versus p210), the bcr-abl fusion gene may be detectable only by pulsed-field gel electrophoresis or reverse-transcriptase polymerase chain reaction (RT-PCR). These tests should be performed whenever possible in patients with ALL, especially those with B-cell lineage disease. Two other chromosomal abnormalities with poor prognoses are t(4;11), which is characterized by rearrangements of the MLL gene and may be rearranged despite normal cytogenetics, and t(9;22). In addition to t(9;22) and t(4;11), patients with deletion of chromosome 7 or trisomy 8 have been reported to have a lower probability of survival at 5 years compared to patients with a normal karyotype.[30] L3 ALL is associated with a variety of translocations which involve translocation of the c-myc proto-oncogene to the immunoglobulin gene locus (t(2;8), t(8;12), and t(8;22)).

Cellular Classification

Leukemic cell characteristics including morphological features, cytochemistry, immunologic cell surface and biochemical markers, and cytogenetic characteristics are important. In adults, FAB L1 morphology (more mature appearing lymphoblasts) is present in fewer than 50% of

[28] Gaynor J, Chapman D, Little C, et al.: A cause-specific hazard rate analysis of prognostic factors among 199 adults with acute lymphoblastic leukemia: the Memorial Hospital experience since 1969. Journal of Clinical Oncology 6(6): 1014-1030, 1988.
Hoelzer D, Thiel E, Loffler H, et al.: Prognostic factors in a multicenter study for treatment of acute lymphoblastic leukemia in adults. Blood 71(1): 123-131, 1988.
[29] Kantarjian HM, Smith T, Estey E, et al.: Prognostic significance of elevated serum beta2-microglobulin levels in adult acute lymphocytic leukemia. American Journal of Medicine 93(6): 599-604, 1992.
[30] Wetzler M, Dodge RK, Mrozek K, et al.: Prospective karyotype analysis in adult acute lymphoblastic leukemia: the Cancer and Leukemia Group B experience. Blood 93(11): 3983-3993, 1999.

patients and L2 histology (more immature and pleomorphic) predominates.[31] Chromosomal abnormalities including aneuploidy and translocations have been described and may correlate with prognosis.[32] In particular, patients with Philadelphia chromosome-positive (Ph+) t(9;22) acute lymphoblastic leukemia (ALL) have a poor prognosis and represent more than 30% of adult cases. The bcr-abl fusion gene resulting from the breakpoint in the Ph chromosome may, on occasion, be detectable only by pulse-field gel electrophoresis or reverse-transcriptase polymerase chain reaction. Bcr-abl rearranged leukemias that do not demonstrate the classical Ph chromosome carry a poor prognosis that is similar to those that are Ph+.

Using heteroantisera and monoclonal antibodies, ALL cells can be divided into early B-cell lineage (80% approximate frequency), T-cells (10%-15% approximate frequency), B cells (with surface immunoglobulins), (<5% approximate frequency), and CALLA+ (common ALL antigen), 50% approximate frequency.[33]

A subset of ALL patients whose blast cells co-expressed myeloid antigens has been described. Complete response rates and overall survival were significantly lower in such patients. These patients tend to be older than other ALL patients. Thus, cytogenetics and immunologic phenotyping may be of great importance in defining prognostic subgroups. Molecular biologic studies that assess the prognostic and diagnostic impact of rearrangements of the immunoglobulin gene and T-cell receptor gene are also in progress.[34]

About 95% of all types of ALL except B cell (which usually has an L3 morphology by the FAB classification) have elevated terminal deoxynucleotidyl transferase (TdT) expression. This elevation is extremely

---

[31] Brearley RL, Johnson SA, Lister TA: Acute lymphoblastic leukaemia in adults: clinicopathological correlations with the French-American-British (FAB) co-operative group classification. European Journal of Cancer 15(6): 909-914, 1979.

[32] Chromosomal abnormalities and their clinical significance in acute lymphoblastic leukemia. Third International Workshop on Chromosomes in Leukemia. Cancer Research 43(2): 868-873, 1983.

[33] Brearley RL, Johnson SA, Lister TA: Acute lymphoblastic leukaemia in adults: clinicopathological correlations with the French-American-British (FAB) co-operative group classification. European Journal of Cancer 15(6): 909-914, 1979.

Hoelzer D, Thiel E, Loffler H, et al.: Prognostic factors in a multicenter study for treatment of acute lymphoblastic leukemia in adults. Blood 71(1): 123-131, 1988.

Sobol RE, Royston I, LeBien TW, et al.: Adult acute lymphoblastic leukemia phenotypes defined by monoclonal antibodies. Blood 65(3): 730-735, 1985.

Foon KA, Billing RJ, Terasaki PI, et al.: Immunologic classification of acute lymphoblastic leukemia implications for normal lymphoid differentiation. Blood 56(6): 1120-1126, 1980.

[34] Davey FR, Mick R, Nelson DA, et al.: Morphologic and cytochemical characterization of adult lymphoid leukemias which express myeloid antigen. Leukemia 2(7): 420-426, 1988.

useful in diagnosis; if concentrations of the enzyme are not elevated, the diagnosis of ALL is suspect. However, 20% of cases of acute myeloid leukemia (AML) may express TdT; therefore, its usefulness as a lineage marker is limited.

Stage Information

There is no clear-cut staging system for this disease.

Untreated

For a newly diagnosed patient with no prior treatment, untreated adult acute lymphoblastic leukemia (ALL) is defined as an abnormal white blood cell count and differential, abnormal hematocrit/hemoglobin and platelet counts, abnormal bone marrow with more than 5% blasts, and signs and symptoms of the disease.

In Remission

A patient who has received remission-induction treatment of ALL is in remission if the bone marrow is normocellular with less than 5% blasts, there are no signs or symptoms of the disease, no signs or symptoms of central nervous system leukemia or other extramedullary infiltration, and all of the following laboratory values are within normal limits: white blood cell count and differential, hematocrit/hemoglobin level, and platelet count.

Treatment Option Overview

Successful treatment of acute lymphoblastic leukemia (ALL) consists of the control of bone marrow and systemic disease as well as the treatment (or prevention) of sanctuary-site disease, particularly the central nervous system (CNS).[35] The cornerstone of this strategy includes systemically administered combination chemotherapy with CNS preventive therapy. CNS prophylaxis

---

[35] Clarkson BD, Gee T, Mertelsmann R, et al.: Current status of treatment of acute leukemia in adults: an overview of the Memorial experience and review of literature. Critical Reviews in Oncology/Hematology 4(3): 221-248, 1986.
Hoelzer D, Gale RP: Acute lymphoblastic leukemia in adults: recent progress, future directions. Seminars in Hematology 24(1): 27-39, 1987.

is achieved with chemotherapy (intrathecal and/or high-dose systemic) and, in some cases, cranial irradiation.

Treatment is divided into 3 phases: remission induction, CNS prophylaxis, and remission continuation or maintenance. The average length of treatment of ALL varies between 1.5 and 3 years in the effort to eradicate the leukemic cell population. Younger adults with ALL may be eligible for selected clinical trials for childhood ALL.

It has been recognized for many years that some patients presenting with acute leukemia may have a cytogenetic abnormality that is morphologically indistinguishable from the Philadelphia (Ph) chromosome.[36] The Ph chromosome occurs in only 1% to 2% of patients with AML, but it occurs in about 20% of adults and a small percentage of children with ALL.[37] In the majority of children and in more than one half of adults with Ph chromosome-positive (Ph+) ALL, the molecular abnormality is different from that in Ph+ chronic myelogenous leukemia (CML).

Ph+ ALL has a worse prognosis than most other types of ALL, although many children and some adults with Ph+ ALL may have complete remissions following intensive ALL treatment clinical trials. If a suitable donor is available, allogeneic bone marrow transplantation should be considered because remissions are generally short with conventional ALL chemotherapy clinical trials. Many patients who have molecular evidence of the bcr-abl fusion gene, which characterizes the Ph chromosome, have no evidence of the abnormal chromosome by cytogenetics. Because many patients have a different fusion protein from the one found in CML (p190 versus p210), the bcr-abl fusion gene may be detectable only by pulsed-field gel electrophoresis or reverse-transcriptase polymerase chain reaction (RT-PCR). These tests should be performed whenever possible in patients with ALL, especially those with B-cell lineage disease. Two other chromosomal abnormalities with poor prognosis are t(4;11), which is characterized by rearrangements of the MLL gene and may be rearranged despite normal cytogenetics, and t(9;22). In addition to t(9;22) and t(4;11), patients with deletion of chromosome 7 or trisomy 8 have been reported to have a lower probability of survival at 5 years compared to patients with a normal karyotype. In multivariate analysis, karyotype was the most important

---

[36] Peterson LC, Bloomfield CD, Brunning RD: Blast crisis as an initial or terminal manifestation of chronic myeloid leukemia: a study of 28 patients. American Journal of Medicine 60(2): 209-220, 1976.

[37] Secker-Walker LM, Cooke HM, Browett PJ, et al.: Variable Philadelphia breakpoints and potential lineage restriction of bcr rearrangement in acute lymphoblastic leukemia. Blood 72(2): 784-791, 1988.

predictor of disease-free survival.[38] [Level of evidence: 3iiDi] L3 ALL is associated with a variety of translocations which involve translocation of the c-myc proto-oncogene to the immunoglobulin gene locus (t(2;8), t(8;12), and t(8;22)). Unlike bcr-abl-positive ALL and t(4;11) ALL, there is some evidence that L3 leukemia can be cured with aggressive, rapidly cycling lymphoma-like chemotherapy regimens.[39]

The designations in PDQ that treatments are "standard" or "under clinical evaluation" are not to be used as a basis for reimbursement determinations.

Untreated Adult Acute Lymphoblastic Leukemia

Standard treatment options for remission induction therapy:

- Most current induction regimens for adult acute lymphoblastic leukemia (ALL) include prednisone, vincristine, and an anthracycline.

- Some regimens also add other drugs, such as asparaginase or cyclophosphamide.

- Current multiagent induction regimens result in complete response rates that range from 60% to 90%.[40]

Two subtypes of adult ALL require special consideration. B-cell ALL [which expresses surface immunoglobulin and cytogenetic abnormalities such as t(8;14), t(2;8), and t(8;22)] is not usually cured with typical ALL regimens. Aggressive cyclophosphamide-based regimens similar to those used in aggressive non-Hodgkin's lymphoma have shown high response rates and cure.[41] T-cell ALL, including lymphoblastic lymphoma, similarly has shown

---

[38] Wetzler M, Dodge RK, Mrozek K, et al.: Prospective karyotype analysis in adult acute lymphoblastic leukemia: the Cancer and Leukemia Group B experience. Blood 93(11): 3983-3993, 1999.

[39] Fenaux P, Lai JL, Miaux O, et al.: Burkitt cell acute leukaemia (L3 ALL) in adults: a report of 18 cases. British Journal of Haematology 71: 371-376, 1989.
Reiter A, Schrappe M, Ludwig W, et al.: Favorable outcome of B-cell acute lymphoblastic leukemia in childhood: a report of three consecutive studies of the BFM Group. Blood 80(10): 2471-2478, 1992.

[40] Hoelzer D, Thiel E, Loffler H, et al.: Prognostic factors in a multicenter study for treatment of acute lymphoblastic leukemia in adults. Blood 71(1): 123-131, 1988.
Linker CA, Levitt LJ, O'Donnell M, et al.: Treatment of adult acute lymphoblastic leukemia with intensive cyclical chemotherapy: a follow-up report. Blood 78(11): 2814-2822, 1991.
Larson RA, Dodge RK, Burns CP, et al.: A five-drug remission induction regimen with intensive consolidation for adults with acute lymphoblastic leukemia: Cancer and Leukemia Group B study 8811. Blood 85(8): 2025-2037, 1995.

[41] Hoelzer D, Ludwig WD, Thiel E, et al.: Improved outcome in adult B-cell acute lymphoblastic leukemia. Blood 87(2): 495-508, 1996.

high cure rates when treated with cyclophosphamide-containing regimens.[42] Whenever possible, such patients should be entered in clinical trials designed to improve the outcomes in these subsets.[43]

Since myelosuppression is an anticipated consequence of both the leukemia and its treatment with chemotherapy, patients must be closely monitored during remission induction treatment. Facilities must be available for hematological support as well as for the treatment of infectious complications.

Supportive care during remission induction treatment should routinely include red blood cell and platelet transfusions when appropriate.[44] Randomized trials have shown similar outcomes for patients who received prophylactic platelet transfusions at a level of 10,000 per cubic millimeter rather than 20,000 per cubic millimeter.[45] The incidence of platelet alloimmunization was similar among groups randomly assigned to receive pooled platelet concentrates from random donors; filtered, pooled platelet concentrates from random donors; ultraviolet B-irradiated, pooled platelet concentrates from random donors; or filtered platelets obtained by apheresis from single random donors.[46] Empiric broad spectrum antimicrobial therapy is an absolute necessity for febrile patients who are profoundly neutropenic.[47] Careful instruction in personal hygiene, dental care, and recognition of early signs of infection are appropriate in all patients. Elaborate isolation facilities, including filtered air, sterile food, and gut flora sterilization are not routinely

---

[42] Larson RA, Dodge RK, Burns CP, et al.: A five-drug remission induction regimen with intensive consolidation for adults with acute lymphoblastic leukemia: Cancer and Leukemia Group B study 8811. Blood 85(8): 2025-2037, 1995.

[43] Refer to the PDQ summary on Adult Non-Hodgkin's Lymphoma Treatment for more information on B-cell (Burkitt's) lymphoma and T-cell (lymphoblastic) lymphoma.

[44] Slichter SJ: Controversies in platelet transfusion therapy. Annual Review of Medicine 31: 509-540, 1980.

Murphy MF, Metcalfe P, Thomas H, et al.: Use of leucocyte-poor blood components and HLA-matched-platelet donors to prevent HLA alloimmunization. British Journal of Haematology 62(3): 529-534, 1986.

[45] Rebulla P, Finazzi G, Marangoni F, et al.: The threshold for prophylactic platelet transfusions in adults with acute myeloid leukemia. New England Journal of Medicine 337(26): 1870-1875, 1997.

[46] The Trial to Reduce Alloimmunization to Platelets Study Group: Leukocyte reduction and ultraviolet B irradiation of platelets to prevent alloimmunization and refractoriness to platelet transfusions. New England Journal of Medicine 337(26): 1861-1869, 1997.

[47] Hughes WT, Armstrong D, Bodey GP, et al.: Guidelines for the use of antimicrobial agents in neutropenic patients with unexplained fever. Journal of Infectious Diseases 161(3): 381-396, 1990.

Rubin M, Hathorn JW, Pizzo PA: Controversies in the management of febrile neutropenic cancer patients. Cancer Investigation 6(2): 167-184, 1988.

indicated but may benefit transplant patients.[48] Rapid marrow ablation with consequent earlier marrow regeneration decreases morbidity and mortality. White blood cell transfusions can be beneficial in selected patients with aplastic marrow and serious infections that are not responding to antibiotics.[49] Prophylactic oral antibiotics may be appropriate in patients with expected prolonged, profound granulocytopenia (<100 per cubic millimeter for 2 weeks), although further studies are necessary.[50] To detect the presence or acquisition of resistant organisms, serial surveillance cultures may be helpful in such patients. The use of myeloid growth factors during remission induction therapy appears to decrease the time to hematopoietic reconstitution.[51]

Treatment options for remission induction therapy under clinical evaluation:

- Clinical trials are ongoing, and patients should be considered for these studies.[52]

The early institution of CNS prophylaxis is critical to achieve control of sanctuary disease. Standard treatment options for central nervous system (CNS) prophylaxis:

- Cranial irradiation plus intrathecal (IT) methotrexate.

- High-dose systemic methotrexate and IT methotrexate without cranial irradiation.

- IT chemotherapy alone.

---

[48] Armstrong, D: Protected environments are discomforting and expensive and do not offer meaningful protection. American Journal of Medicine 76: 685-689, 1984.
Sherertz RJ, Belani A, Kramer BS, et al.: Impact of air filtration on nosocomial Aspergillus infections: unique risk of bone marrow transplant recipients. American Journal of Medicine 83(4): 709-718, 1987.
[49] Schiffer CA: Granulocyte transfusions: an overlooked therapeutic modality. Transfusion Medicine Reviews 4(1): 2-7, 1990.
[50] Wade JC, Schimpff SC, Hargadon MT, et al.: A comparison of trimethoprim-sulfamethoxazole plus nystatin with gentamicin plus nystatin in the prevention of infections in acute leukemia. New England Journal of Medicine 304(18): 1057-1062, 1981.
[51] Scherrer R, Geissler K, Kyrle PA, et al.: Granulocyte colony-stimulating factor (G-CSF) as an adjunct to induction chemotherapy of adult acute lymphoblastic leukemia (ALL). Annals of Hematology 66(6): 283-289, 1993.
Larson RA, Dodge RK, Linker CA, et al.: A randomized controlled trial of filgrastim during remssion induction and consolidation chemotherapy for adults with acute lymphoblastic leukemia: CALGB study 9111. Blood 92(5): 1556-1564, 1998.
[52] Radford JE, Burns CP, Jones MP, et al.: Adult acute lymphoblastic leukemia: results of the Iowa HOP-L protocol. Journal of Clinical Oncology 7(1): 58-66, 1989.

Adult Acute Lymphoblastic Leukemia in Remission

Current approaches to postremission therapy for adult acute lymphoblastic leukemia (ALL) include short-term, relatively intensive chemotherapy followed by longer-term therapy at lower doses (maintenance), high-dose marrow-ablative chemotherapy or chemoradiotherapy with allogeneic stem cell rescue (alloBMT), and high-dose therapy with autologous stem cell rescue (autoBMT). Several trials of aggressive postremission chemotherapy for adult ALL now confirm a long-term disease-free survival rate of approximately 40%.[53] In the latter 2 series, especially good prognoses were found for patients with T-cell lineage ALL, with disease-free survival rates of 50% to 70% for patients receiving postremission therapy. These series represent a significant improvement in disease-free survival rates over previous, less intensive chemotherapeutic approaches. In contrast, poor cure rates were demonstrated in patients with Philadelphia chromosome-positive (Ph+) ALL, B-cell lineage ALL with an L3 phenotype (surface immunoglobulin positive), and B-cell lineage ALL characterized by t(4;11). Administration of the newer dose-intensive schedules can be difficult and should be performed by physicians experienced in these regimens at centers equipped to deal with potential complications. Studies in which continuation or maintenance chemotherapy were eliminated had outcomes inferior to those with extended treatment durations.[54]

AlloBMT results in the lowest incidence of leukemic relapse, even when compared with a bone marrow transplant from an identical twin (syngeneic BMT). This finding has led to the concept of an immunologic graft-versus-

---

[53] Gaynor J, Chapman D, Little C, et al.: A cause-specific hazard rate analysis of prognostic factors among 199 adults with acute lymphoblastic leukemia: the Memorial Hospital experience since 1969. Journal of Clinical Oncology 6(6): 1014-1030, 1988.

Hoelzer D, Thiel E, Loffler H, et al.: Prognostic factors in a multicenter study for treatment of acute lymphoblastic leukemia in adults. Blood 71(1): 123-131, 1988.

Linker CA, Levitt LJ, O'Donnell M, et al.: Treatment of adult acute lymphoblastic leukemia with intensive cyclical chemotherapy: a follow-up report. Blood 78(11): 2814-2822, 1991.

Zhang MJ, Hoelzer D, Horowitz MM, et al.: Long-term follow-up of adults with acute lymphoblastic leukemia in first remission treated with chemotherapy or bone marrow transplantation. Annals of Internal Medicine 123(6): 428-431, 1995.

Larson RA, Dodge RK, Burns CP, et al.: A five-drug remission induction regimen with intensive consolidation for adults with acute lymphoblastic leukemia: Cancer and Leukemia Group B study 8811. Blood 85(8): 2025-2037, 1995.

[54] Cuttner J, Mick R, Budman DR, et al.: Phase III trial of brief intensive treatment of adult acute lymphocytic leukemia comparing daunorubicin and mitoxantrone: a CALGB study. Leukemia 5(5): 425-431, 1991.

Dekker AW, van't Veer MB, Sizoo W, et al.: Intensive postremission chemotherapy without maintenance therapy in adults with acute lymphoblastic leukemia. Journal of Clinical Oncology 15(2): 476-482, 1997.

leukemia effect similar to graft-versus-host disease (GVHD). The improvement in disease-free survival in patients undergoing alloBMT as primary postremission therapy is offset, in part, by the increased morbidity and mortality from GVHD, veno-occlusive disease of the liver, and interstitial pneumonitis.[55] The results of a retrospective study showed a similar outcome to that for intensive chemotherapy for patients receiving alloBMT in first remission in both the International Bone Marrow Transplant Registry and the German chemotherapy trial (Berlin-Frankfurt-Munster).[56] In a prospective French trial, adults with ALL in remission and who were younger than age 40 years received alloBMT if a sibling donor was available or were randomly assigned to either ongoing chemotherapy or autoBMT. There was no advantage to alloBMT for the group of patients with standard-risk ALL.[57] There was, however, significant survival benefit to alloBMT for patients with high-risk ALL (CD10-; B-cell lineage ALL with a white blood cell count >30,000; Ph1+ ALL). This trial confirms the experience of a single institution that suggested the utility of alloBMT for the cure of high-risk ALL.[58] The long-term survival of patients in the French randomized study who received chemotherapy and autoBMT was identical.[59] The use of alloBMT as primary postremission therapy is limited both by the need for an HLA-matched sibling donor and by the increased mortality from alloBMT in patients in their 5th or 6th decade. The mortality from alloBMT using an HLA-matched sibling donor ranges from 20% to 40%, depending on the study. The use of matched unrelated donors for alloBMT is currently under evaluation but, because of its current high treatment-related morbidity and mortality, is reserved for patients in second remission or beyond. The dose of total body irradiation administered is associated with the incidence of acute and chronic GVHD and may be an independent predictor of leukemia-free survival.[60] [Level of evidence: 3iiB]

---

[55] Finiewicz KJ, Larson RA: Dose-intensive therapy for adult acute lymphoblastic leukemia. Seminars in Oncology 26(1): 6-20, 1999.

[56] Horowitz MM, Messerer D, Hoelzer D, et al.: Chemotherapy compared with bone marrow transplantation for adults with acute lymphoblastic leukemia in first remission. Annals of Internal Medicine 115(1): 13-18, 1991.

[57] Sebban C, Lepage E, Vernant J, et al.: Allogeneic bone marrow transplantation in adult acute lymphoblastic leukemia in first complete remission: a comparative study. Journal of Clinical Oncology 12(12): 2580-2587, 1994.

[58] Forman SJ, O'Donnell MR, Nademanee AP, et al.: Bone marrow transplantation for patients with Philadelphia chromosome-positive acute lymphoblastic leukemia. Blood 70(2): 587-588, 1987.

[59] Fiere D, Lepage E, Sebban C, et al.: Adult acute lymphoblastic leukemia: a multicentric randomized trial testing bone marrow transplantation as postremission therapy. Journal of Clinical Oncology 11(10): 1990-2001, 1993.

[60] Corvo R, Paoli G, Barra S, et al.: Total body irradiation correlates with chronic graft versus host disease and affects prognosis of patients with acute lymphoblastic leukemia receiving

Aggressive cyclophosphamide-based regimens similar to those used in aggressive non-Hodgkin's lymphoma have shown improved outcome of prolonged disease-free status for patients with B-cell ALL (L3 morphology, surface immunoglobulin positive).[61] Retrospectively reviewing 3 sequential cooperative group trials from Germany, Hoelzer and colleagues found a marked improvement in survival, from zero survivors in a 1981 study that used standard pediatric therapy and lasted 2.5 years, to a 50% survival rate in 2 subsequent trials that used rapidly alternating lymphoma-like chemotherapy and were completed within 6 months. Aggressive CNS prophylaxis remains a prominent component of treatment. This report, which requires confirmation in other cooperative group settings, is encouraging for patients with L3 ALL. Patients with surface immunoglobulin but L1 or L2 morphology did not benefit from this regimen. Similarly, patients with L3 morphology and immunophenotype but unusual cytogenetic features were not cured with this approach. A white blood cell count of less than 50,000 per microliter predicted improved leukemia-free survival in univariate analysis. Because the optimal postremission therapy for patients with ALL is still unclear, participation in clinical trials should be considered.

The early institution of CNS prophylaxis is critical to achieve control of sanctuary disease. Some authors have suggested that there is a subgroup of patients at low-risk for CNS relapse for whom CNS prophylaxis may not be necessary. However, this concept has not been tested prospectively.[62]

Standard treatment options for central nervous system (CNS) prophylaxis:

- Cranial irradiation plus intrathecal (IT) methotrexate.

- High-dose systemic methotrexate and IT methotrexate without cranial irradiation.

- IT chemotherapy alone.

---

an HLA identical allogeneic bone marrow transplant. International Journal of Radiation Oncology, Biology, Physics 43(3): 497-503, 1999.

[61] Hoelzer D, Ludwig WD, Thiel E, et al.: Improved outcome in adult B-cell acute lymphoblastic leukemia. Blood 87(2): 495-508, 1996.

[62] Kantarjian HM, Walters RS, Smith TL, et al.: Identification of risk groups for development of central nervous system leukemia in adults with acute lymphocytic leukemia. Blood 72(5): 1784-1789, 1988.

Recurrent Adult Acute Lymphoblastic Leukemia

Patients who experience a relapse following chemotherapy and maintenance therapy are unlikely to be cured by further chemotherapy alone. These patients should be considered for reinduction chemotherapy followed by allogeneic bone marrow transplantation. Patients for whom an HLA-matched donor is not available are excellent candidates for enrollment in clinical trials that are studying autologous transplantation, immunomodulation, and novel chemotherapeutic or biological agents.[63] Low-dose palliative radiation therapy may be considered in patients with symptomatic recurrence either within or outside the central nervous system.[64]

For More Information

About PDQ

- **PDQ® - NCI's Comprehensive Cancer Database.**
  Full description of the NCI PDQ database.

Additional PDQ Summaries

- **PDQ® Cancer Information Summaries: Adult Treatment**
  Treatment options for adult cancers.

---

[63] Herzig RH, Barrett AJ, Gluckman E, et al.: Bone-marrow transplantation in high-risk acute lymphoblastic leukaemia in first and second remission. Lancet 1(8536): 786-789, 1987.
Thomas ED, Sanders JE, Flournoy N, et al.: Marrow transplantation for patients with acute lymphoblastic leukemia: a long-term follow-up. Blood 62(5): 1139-1141, 1983.
Barrett AJ, Horowitz MM, Gale RP, et al.: Marrow transplantation for acute lymphoblastic leukemia: factors affecting relapse and survival. Blood 74(2): 862-871, 1989.
Dinsmore R, Kirkpatrick D, Flomenberg N, et al.: Allogeneic bone marrow transplantation for patients with acute lymphoblastic leukemia. Blood 62(2): 381-388, 1983.
Sallan SE, Niemeyer CM, Billett AL, et al.: Autologous bone marrow transplantation for acute lymphoblastic leukemia. Journal of Clinical Oncology 7(11): 1594-1601, 1989.
Paciucci PA, Keaveney C, Cuttner J, et al.: Mitoxantrone, vincristine and prednisone in adults with relapsed or primarily refractory acute lymphocytic leukemia and terminal deoxynucleotidyl transferase positive blastic phase of chronic myelocytic leukemia. Cancer Research 47(19): 5234-5237, 1987.
Biggs JC, Horowitz MM, Gale RP, et al.: Bone marrow transplants may cure patients with acute leukemia never achieving remission with chemotherapy. Blood 80(4): 1090-1093, 1992.
[64] Gray JR, Wallner KE: Reversal of cranial nerve dysfunction with radiation therapy in adults with lymphoma and leukemia. International Journal of Radiation Oncology, Biology, Physics 19(2): 439-444, 1990.

- **PDQ® Cancer Information Summaries: Pediatric Treatment**
Treatment options for childhood cancers.

- **PDQ® Cancer Information Summaries: Supportive Care**
Side effects of cancer treatment, management of cancer-related complications and pain, and psychosocial concerns.

- **PDQ® Cancer Information Summaries: Screening/Detection (Testing for Cancer)**
Tests or procedures that detect specific types of cancer.

- **PDQ® Cancer Information Summaries: Prevention**
Risk factors and methods to increase chances of preventing specific types of cancer.

- **PDQ® Cancer Information Summaries: Genetics**
Genetics of specific cancers and inherited cancer syndromes, and ethical, legal, and social concerns.

- **PDQ® Cancer Information Summaries: Complementary and Alternative Medicine**
Information about complementary and alternative forms of treatment for patients with cancer.

NIH Databases

In addition to the various Institutes of Health that publish professional guidelines, the NIH has designed a number of databases for professionals.[65] Physician-oriented resources provide a wide variety of information related to the biomedical and health sciences, both past and present. The format of these resources varies. Searchable databases, bibliographic citations, full text articles (when available), archival collections, and images are all available. The following are referenced by the National Library of Medicine:[66]

- **Bioethics:** Access to published literature on the ethical, legal and public policy issues surrounding healthcare and biomedical research. This information is provided in conjunction with the Kennedy Institute of Ethics located at Georgetown University, Washington, D.C.: **http://www.nlm.nih.gov/databases/databases_bioethics.html**

---

[65] Remember, for the general public, the National Library of Medicine recommends the databases referenced in MEDLINE*plus* (**http://medlineplus.gov/** or **http://www.nlm.nih.gov/medlineplus/databases.html**).
[66] See **http://www.nlm.nih.gov/databases/databases.html**.

- **HIV/AIDS Resources:** Describes various links and databases dedicated to HIV/AIDS research: http://www.nlm.nih.gov/pubs/factsheets/aidsinfs.html

- **NLM Online Exhibitions:** Describes "Exhibitions in the History of Medicine": http://www.nlm.nih.gov/exhibition/exhibition.html. Additional resources for historical scholarship in medicine: http://www.nlm.nih.gov/hmd/hmd.html

- **Biotechnology Information:** Access to public databases. The National Center for Biotechnology Information conducts research in computational biology, develops software tools for analyzing genome data, and disseminates biomedical information for the better understanding of molecular processes affecting human health and disease: http://www.ncbi.nlm.nih.gov/

- **Population Information:** The National Library of Medicine provides access to worldwide coverage of population, family planning, and related health issues, including family planning technology and programs, fertility, and population law and policy: http://www.nlm.nih.gov/databases/databases_population.html

- **Cancer Information:** Access to caner-oriented databases: http://www.nlm.nih.gov/databases/databases_cancer.html

- **Profiles in Science:** Offering the archival collections of prominent twentieth-century biomedical scientists to the public through modern digital technology: http://www.profiles.nlm.nih.gov/

- **Chemical Information:** Provides links to various chemical databases and references: http://sis.nlm.nih.gov/Chem/ChemMain.html

- **Clinical Alerts:** Reports the release of findings from the NIH-funded clinical trials where such release could significantly affect morbidity and mortality: http://www.nlm.nih.gov/databases/alerts/clinical_alerts.html

- **Space Life Sciences:** Provides links and information to space-based research (including NASA): http://www.nlm.nih.gov/databases/databases_space.html

- **MEDLINE:** Bibliographic database covering the fields of medicine, nursing, dentistry, veterinary medicine, the healthcare system, and the pre-clinical sciences: http://www.nlm.nih.gov/databases/databases_medline.html

- **Toxicology and Environmental Health Information (TOXNET):** Databases covering toxicology and environmental health: http://sis.nlm.nih.gov/Tox/ToxMain.html

- **Visible Human Interface:** Anatomically detailed, three-dimensional representations of normal male and female human bodies: **http://www.nlm.nih.gov/research/visible/visible_human.html**

While all of the above references may be of interest to physicians who study and treat adult acute lymphoblastic leukemia, the following are particularly noteworthy.

The NLM Gateway[67]

The NLM (National Library of Medicine) Gateway is a Web-based system that lets users search simultaneously in multiple retrieval systems at the U.S. National Library of Medicine (NLM). It allows users of NLM services to initiate searches from one Web interface, providing "one-stop searching" for many of NLM's information resources or databases.[68] One target audience for the Gateway is the Internet user who is new to NLM's online resources and does not know what information is available or how best to search for it. This audience may include physicians and other healthcare providers, researchers, librarians, students, and, increasingly, patients, their families, and the public.[69] To use the NLM Gateway, simply go to the search site at **http://gateway.nlm.nih.gov/gw/Cmd**. Type "adult acute lymphoblastic leukemia" (or synonyms) into the search box and click "Search." The results will be presented in a tabular form, indicating the number of references in each database category.

---

[67] Adapted from NLM: **http://gateway.nlm.nih.gov/gw/Cmd?Overview.x**.

[68] The NLM Gateway is currently being developed by the Lister Hill National Center for Biomedical Communications (LHNCBC) at the National Library of Medicine (NLM) of the National Institutes of Health (NIH).

[69] Other users may find the Gateway useful for an overall search of NLM's information resources. Some searchers may locate what they need immediately, while others will utilize the Gateway as an adjunct tool to other NLM search services such as PubMed® and MEDLINEplus®. The Gateway connects users with multiple NLM retrieval systems while also providing a search interface for its own collections. These collections include various types of information that do not logically belong in PubMed, LOCATORplus, or other established NLM retrieval systems (e.g., meeting announcements and pre-1966 journal citations). The Gateway will provide access to the information found in an increasing number of NLM retrieval systems in several phases.

Results Summary

Category	Items Found
Journal Articles	16397
Books / Periodicals / Audio Visual	33
Consumer Health	806
Meeting Abstracts	7
Other Collections	103
Total	17346

HSTAT[70]

HSTAT is a free, Web-based resource that provides access to full-text documents used in healthcare decision-making.[71] HSTAT's audience includes healthcare providers, health service researchers, policy makers, insurance companies, consumers, and the information professionals who serve these groups. HSTAT provides access to a wide variety of publications, including clinical practice guidelines, quick-reference guides for clinicians, consumer health brochures, evidence reports and technology assessments from the Agency for Healthcare Research and Quality (AHRQ), as well as AHRQ's Put Prevention Into Practice.[72] Simply search by "adult acute lymphoblastic leukemia" (or synonyms) at the following Web site: **http://text.nlm.nih.gov**.

Coffee Break: Tutorials for Biologists[73]

Some patients may wish to have access to a general healthcare site that takes a scientific view of the news and covers recent breakthroughs in biology that may one day assist physicians in developing treatments. To this end, we recommend "Coffee Break," a collection of short reports on recent biological

---

[70] Adapted from HSTAT: **http://www.nlm.nih.gov/pubs/factsheets/hstat.html**.

[71] The HSTAT URL is **http://hstat.nlm.nih.gov/**.

[72] Other important documents in HSTAT include: the National Institutes of Health (NIH) Consensus Conference Reports and Technology Assessment Reports; the HIV/AIDS Treatment Information Service (ATIS) resource documents; the Substance Abuse and Mental Health Services Administration's Center for Substance Abuse Treatment (SAMHSA/CSAT) Treatment Improvement Protocols (TIP) and Center for Substance Abuse Prevention (SAMHSA/CSAP) Prevention Enhancement Protocols System (PEPS); the Public Health Service (PHS) Preventive Services Task Force's *Guide to Clinical Preventive Services*; the independent, nonfederal Task Force on Community Services *Guide to Community Preventive Services*; and the Health Technology Advisory Committee (HTAC) of the Minnesota Health Care Commission (MHCC) health technology evaluations.

[73] Adapted from **http://www.ncbi.nlm.nih.gov/Coffeebreak/Archive/FAQ.html**.

discoveries. Each report incorporates interactive tutorials that demonstrate how bioinformatics tools are used as a part of the research process. Currently, all Coffee Breaks are written by NCBI staff.[74] Each report is about 400 words and is usually based on a discovery reported in one or more articles from recently published, peer-reviewed literature.[75] This site has new articles every few weeks, so it can be considered an online magazine of sorts, and intended for general background information. You can access Coffee Break at **http://www.ncbi.nlm.nih.gov/Coffeebreak/**.

Other Commercial Databases

In addition to resources maintained by official agencies, other databases exist that are commercial ventures addressing medical professionals. Here are some examples that may interest you:

- **CliniWeb International:** Index and table of contents to selected clinical information on the Internet; see **http://www.ohsu.edu/cliniweb/**.

- **Medical World Search:** Searches full text from thousands of selected medical sites on the Internet; see **http://www.mwsearch.com/**.

---

[74] The figure that accompanies each article is frequently supplied by an expert external to NCBI, in which case the source of the figure is cited. The result is an interactive tutorial that tells a biological story.

[75] After a brief introduction that sets the work described into a broader context, the report focuses on how a molecular understanding can provide explanations of observed biology and lead to therapies for diseases. Each vignette is accompanied by a figure and hypertext links that lead to a series of pages that interactively show how NCBI tools and resources are used in the research process.

CHAPTER 6. DISSERTATIONS ON ADULT ACUTE LYMPHOBLASTIC LEUKEMIA

Overview

University researchers are active in studying almost all known diseases. The result of research is often published in the form of Doctoral or Master's dissertations. You should understand, therefore, that applied diagnostic procedures and/or therapies can take many years to develop after the thesis that proposed the new technique or approach was written.

In this chapter, we will give you a bibliography on recent dissertations relating to adult acute lymphoblastic leukemia. You can read about these in more detail using the Internet or your local medical library. We will also provide you with information on how to use the Internet to stay current on dissertations.

Dissertations on Adult Acute Lymphoblastic Leukemia

ProQuest Digital Dissertations is the largest archive of academic dissertations available. From this archive, we have compiled the following list covering dissertations devoted to adult acute lymphoblastic leukemia. You will see that the information provided includes the dissertation's title, its author, and the author's institution. To read more about the following, simply use the Internet address indicated. The following covers recent dissertations dealing with adult acute lymphoblastic leukemia:

- **Generation and characterization of dendritic-like cells derived from translocation (9;22) acute lymphoblastic leukemia blasts** by Lee, Jaewoo, PhD from State University of New York at Buffalo, 2004, 148 pages
  http://wwwlib.umi.com/dissertations/fullcit/3125732

Keeping Current

As previously mentioned, an effective way to stay current on dissertations dedicated to adult acute lymphoblastic leukemia is to use the database called *ProQuest Digital Dissertations* via the Internet, located at the following Web address: **http://wwwlib.umi.com/dissertations.** The site allows you to freely access the last two years of citations and abstracts. Ask your medical librarian if the library has full and unlimited access to this database. From the library, you should be able to do more complete searches than with the limited 2-year access available to the general public.

Vocabulary Builder

The following vocabulary builder provides definitions of words used in this chapter that have not been defined in previous chapters:

Ablation: The removal of an organ by surgery. [NIH]

Antibiotic: A substance usually produced by vegetal micro-organisms capable of inhibiting the growth of or killing bacteria. [NIH]

Apheresis: Components being separated out, as leukapheresis, plasmapheresis, plateletpheresis. [NIH]

Transcriptase: An enzyme which catalyses the synthesis of a complementary mRNA molecule from a DNA template in the presence of a mixture of the four ribonucleotides (ATP, UTP, GTP and CTP). [NIH]

PART III. APPENDICES

ABOUT PART III

Part III is a collection of appendices on general medical topics which may be of interest to patients with adult acute lymphoblastic leukemia and related conditions.

APPENDIX A. RESEARCHING YOUR MEDICATIONS

Overview

There are a number of sources available on new or existing medications which could be prescribed to patients with adult acute lymphoblastic leukemia. While a number of hard copy or CD-Rom resources are available to patients and physicians for research purposes, a more flexible method is to use Internet-based databases. In this chapter, we will begin with a general overview of medications. We will then proceed to outline official recommendations on how you should view your medications. You may also want to research medications that you are currently taking for other conditions as they may interact with medications for adult acute lymphoblastic leukemia. Research can give you information on the side effects, interactions, and limitations of prescription drugs used in the treatment of adult acute lymphoblastic leukemia. Broadly speaking, there are two sources of information on approved medications: public sources and private sources. We will emphasize free-to-use public sources.

Your Medications: The Basics[76]

The Agency for Health Care Research and Quality has published extremely useful guidelines on how you can best participate in the medication aspects of adult acute lymphoblastic leukemia. Taking medicines is not always as simple as swallowing a pill. It can involve many steps and decisions each day. The AHCRQ recommends that patients with adult acute lymphoblastic leukemia take part in treatment decisions. Do not be afraid to ask questions and talk about your concerns. By taking a moment to ask questions early,

---

[76] This section is adapted from AHCRQ: http://www.ahcpr.gov/consumer/ncpiebro.htm.

you may avoid problems later. Here are some points to cover each time a new medicine is prescribed:

- Ask about all parts of your treatment, including diet changes, exercise, and medicines.

- Ask about the risks and benefits of each medicine or other treatment you might receive.

- Ask how often you or your doctor will check for side effects from a given medication.

Do not hesitate to ask what is important to you about your medicines. You may want a medicine with the fewest side effects, or the fewest doses to take each day. You may care most about cost, or how the medicine might affect how you live or work. Or, you may want the medicine your doctor believes will work the best. Telling your doctor will help him or her select the best treatment for you.

Do not be afraid to "bother" your doctor with your concerns and questions about medications for adult acute lymphoblastic leukemia. You can also talk to a nurse or a pharmacist. They can help you better understand your treatment plan. Feel free to bring a friend or family member with you when you visit your doctor. Talking over your options with someone you trust can help you make better choices, especially if you are not feeling well. Specifically, ask your doctor the following:

- The name of the medicine and what it is supposed to do.

- How and when to take the medicine, how much to take, and for how long.

- What food, drinks, other medicines, or activities you should avoid while taking the medicine.

- What side effects the medicine may have, and what to do if they occur.

- If you can get a refill, and how often.

- About any terms or directions you do not understand.

- What to do if you miss a dose.

- If there is written information you can take home (most pharmacies have information sheets on your prescription medicines; some even offer large-print or Spanish versions).

Do not forget to tell your doctor about all the medicines you are currently taking (not just those for adult acute lymphoblastic leukemia). This includes prescription medicines and the medicines that you buy over the counter. Then your doctor can avoid giving you a new medicine that may not work well with the medications you take now. When talking to your doctor, you may wish to prepare a list of medicines you currently take, the reason you take them, and how you take them. Be sure to include the following information for each:

- Name of medicine

- Reason taken

- Dosage

- Time(s) of day

Also include any over-the-counter medicines, such as:

- Laxatives

- Diet pills

- Vitamins

- Cold medicine

- Aspirin or other pain, headache, or fever medicine

- Cough medicine

- Allergy relief medicine

- Antacids

- Sleeping pills

- Others (include names)

Learning More about Your Medications

Because of historical investments by various organizations and the emergence of the Internet, it has become rather simple to learn about the medications your doctor has recommended for adult acute lymphoblastic leukemia. One such source is the United States Pharmacopeia. In 1820, eleven physicians met in Washington, D.C. to establish the first compendium of standard drugs for the United States. They called this compendium the "U.S. Pharmacopeia (USP)." Today, the USP is a non-profit organization consisting of 800 volunteer scientists, eleven elected officials, and 400 representatives of state associations and colleges of medicine and pharmacy. The USP is located in Rockville, Maryland, and its home page is located at **www.usp.org**. The USP currently provides standards for over 3,700 medications. The resulting USP DI® Advice for the Patient® can be accessed through the National Library of Medicine of the National Institutes of Health. The database is partially derived from lists of federally approved medications in the Food and Drug Administration's (FDA) Drug Approvals database.[77]

While the FDA database is rather large and difficult to navigate, the Phamacopeia is both user-friendly and free to use. It covers more than 9,000 prescription and over-the-counter medications. To access this database, simply type the following hyperlink into your Web browser: **http://www.nlm.nih.gov/medlineplus/druginformation.html**. To view examples of a given medication (brand names, category, description, preparation, proper use, precautions, side effects, etc.), simply follow the hyperlinks indicated within the United States Pharmacopeia (USP).

Of course, we as editors cannot be certain as to what medications you are taking. Therefore, we have compiled a list of medications associated with the treatment of adult acute lymphoblastic leukemia. Once again, due to space limitations, we only list a sample of medications and provide hyperlinks to ample documentation (e.g. typical dosage, side effects, drug-interaction risks, etc.). The following drugs have been mentioned in the Pharmacopeia and other sources as being potentially applicable to adult acute lymphoblastic leukemia:

Teniposide
- **Systemic - U.S. Brands:** Vumon
  http://www.nlm.nih.gov/medlineplus/druginfo/uspdi/203661.html

Commercial Databases

In addition to the medications listed in the USP above, a number of commercial sites are available by subscription to physicians and their institutions. You may be able to access these sources from your local medical library or your doctor's office.

[77] Though cumbersome, the FDA database can be freely browsed at the following site: **www.fda.gov/cder/da/da.htm**.

Reuters Health Drug Database

The Reuters Health Drug Database can be searched by keyword at the hyperlink: **http://www.reutershealth.com/frame2/drug.html**.

Mosby's GenRx

Mosby's GenRx database (also available on CD-Rom and book format) covers 45,000 drug products including generics and international brands. It provides prescribing information, drug interactions, and patient information. Information can be obtained at the following hyperlink: **http://www.genrx.com/Mosby/PhyGenRx/group.html**.

PDR*health*

The PDR*health* database is a free-to-use, drug information search engine that has been written for the public in layman's terms. It contains FDA-approved drug information adapted from the Physicians' Desk Reference (PDR) database. PDR*health* can be searched by brand name, generic name, or indication. It features multiple drug interactions reports. Search PDR*health* at **http://www.pdrhealth.com/drug_info/index.html**.

Other Web Sites

A number of additional Web sites discuss drug information. As an example, you may like to look at **www.drugs.com** which reproduces the information in the Pharmacopeia as well as commercial information. You may also want to consider the Web site of the Medical Letter, Inc. which allows users to download articles on various drugs and therapeutics for a nominal fee: **http://www.medletter.com/**.

Drug Development and Approval

The following Web sites can be valuable resources when conducting research on the development and approval of new cancer drugs:

- FDA Home Page: Search for drugs currently in development or those which have been recently approved by the FDA.
  http://www.fda.gov/

- Cancer Liaison Program: Answers questions from the public about drug approval processes, cancer clinical trials, and access to investigational therapies.
  http://www.fda.gov/oashi/cancer/cancer.html

- Center for Drug Evaluation and Research
  http://www.fda.gov/cder/

- Drug Approvals by Cancer Indications (Alphabetical List)
  http://www.fda.gov/oashi/cancer/cdrugalpha.html

- Drug Approvals by Cancer Indications (Cancer Type)
  http://www.fda.gov/oashi/cancer/cdrugind.html

- Electronic Orange Book of Approved Drug Products
  http://www.fda.gov/cder/ob/default.htm

- Guidance Documents for Industry: Contains an archive of documents describing FDA policies on specific topics.
  http://www.fda.gov/cder/guidance/index.htm

- Industry Collaboration: Provides information to industry on the process for getting new drugs into clinical trials.
  http://ctep.cancer.gov/industry/index.html

- Investigator's Handbook: Provides information to investigators on specific procedures related to clinical trial development.
  http://ctep.cancer.gov/handbook/index.html

- Questions and Answers About NCI's Natural Products Branch: A fact sheet that describes the functions of this branch, which collects and analyzes specimens of plant, marine, and microbial origin for possible anticancer properties.
  http://cis.nci.nih.gov/fact/7_33.htm

Understanding the Approval Process for New Cancer Drugs[78]

Since June 1996, about 80 new cancer-related drugs, or new uses for drugs already on the market, have been approved by the U.S. Food and Drug Administration (FDA), the division of the U.S. Department of Health and Human Services charged with ensuring the safety and effectiveness of new drugs before they can go on the market. (The FDA maintains an annotated online list of drugs approved for use with cancer since 1996.) Some of these

---

[78] Adapted from the NCI:
http://www.cancer.gov/clinical_trials/doc_header.aspx?viewid=d94cbfac-e478-4704-9052-d8e8a3372b56.

drugs treat cancer, some alleviate pain and other symptoms, and, in one case, reduce the risk of invasive cancer in people who are considered high-risk. The FDA relied on the results of clinical trials in making every one of these approvals. Without reliable information about a drug's effects on humans, it would be impossible to approve any drug for widespread use.

When considering a new drug, the FDA faces two challenges:

- First, making sure that the drug is safe and effective before it is made widely available.

- Second, ensuring that drugs which show promise are made available as quickly as possible to the people they can help.

To deal with these challenges, the FDA maintains a rigorous review process but also has measures in place to make some drugs available in special cases. This aim of this section is to acquaint you with the drug approval process and point you to other resources for learning more about it.

The Role of the Federal Drug Administration (FDA)

Approval is only one step in the drug development process. In fact, the FDA estimates that, on average, it takes eight and a half years to study and test a new drug before it can be approved for the general public. That includes early laboratory and animal testing, as well as the clinical trials that evaluate the drugs in humans. The FDA plays a key role at three main points in this process:

- Determining whether or not a new drug shows enough promise to be given to people in clinical trials

- Once clinical trials begin, deciding whether or not they should continue, based on reports of efficacy and adverse reactions

- When clinical trials are completed, deciding whether or not the drug can be sold to the public and what its label should say about directions for use, side effects, warnings, and the like.

To make these decisions, the FDA must review studies submitted by the drug's sponsor (usually the manufacturer), evaluate any adverse reports from preclinical studies and clinical trials (that is, reports of side effects or complications), and review the adequacy of the chemistry and manufacturing. This process is lengthy, but it is meant to ensure that only beneficial drugs with acceptable side effects will make their way into the hands of the public. At the same time, recent legislative mandates and streamlined procedures within the FDA have accelerated the approval of effective drugs, especially for serious illnesses such as cancer. In addition, specific provisions make some drugs available to patients with special needs even before the approval process is complete.

From Lab to Patient Care

By law, the Food and Drug Administration (FDA) must review all test results for new drugs to ensure that products are safe and effective for specific uses. "Safe" does not mean that the drug is free of possible adverse side effects; rather, it means that the potential benefits have been determined to outweigh any risks. The testing process begins long before the first person takes the drug, with preliminary research and animal testing.

If a drug proves promising in the lab, the drug company or sponsor must apply for FDA approval to test it in clinical trials involving people. For drugs, the application, called an Investigational New Drug (IND) Application, is sent through the Center for Drug Evaluation and Research's (CDER) IND Review Process; for biological agents, the IND is sent to the Center for Biologics Evaluation and Research (CBER). Once the IND is approved by CDER or CBER, clinical trials can begin.

If the drug makes it through the clinical trials process—that is, the studies show that it is superior to current drugs—the manufacturer must submit a New Drug Application (NDA) or (for biological agents) a Biologics License Application (BLA) to the FDA. (Biological agents, such as serums, vaccines, and cloned proteins, are manufactured from substances taken from living humans or animals.) This application must include:

- The exact chemical makeup of the drug or biologic and the mechanisms by which it is effective

- Results of animal studies

- Results of clinical trials

- How the drug or biologic is manufactured, processed, and packaged

- Quality control standards

- Samples of the product in the form(s) in which it is to be administered.

Once the FDA receives the NDA or BLA from the manufacturer or developer, the formal New Drug Application Review Process or Biologics/Product License Application Review Process begins.

For an overview of the entire process from start to finish, see the CDER's visual representation of The New Drug Development Process: Steps from Test Tube to New Drug Application Review, which is available for public viewing at **http://www.fda.gov/cder/handbook/develop.htm**.

Speed versus Safety in the Approval Process

The FDA's current goal is that no more than ten months will pass between the time that a complete application is submitted and the FDA takes action on it. But the process is not always smooth. Sometimes FDA's external advisory panels call for additional research or data. In other cases, the FDA staff asks for more information or revised studies. Some new drug approvals have taken as little as 42 days; other more difficult NDAs have spent years in the approval process.

Setting Priorities

The order in which NDAs are assessed by the FDA is determined by a classification system designed to give priority to drugs with the greatest potential benefits. All drugs that offer significant medical advances over existing therapies for any disease are considered "priority" drugs in the approval process. NDAs for cancer treatment drugs are reviewed for this status primarily by the Division of Oncology Drug Products in the FDA's Center for Drug Evaluation and Research (CDER). For Biologic License Applications (vaccines, blood products, and medicines made from animal products), the Center for Biologics Evaluation and Research (CBER) provides additional regulation and oversight.

Expert Advice

The FDA relies on a system of independent advisory committees, made up of professionals from outside the agency, for expert advice and guidance in making sound decisions about drug approval. Each committee meets as needed to weigh available evidence and assess the safety, effectiveness, and appropriate use of products considered for approval. In addition, these committees provide advice about general criteria for evaluation and scientific issues not related to specific products. The Oncologic Drugs Advisory Committee (ODAC) meets regularly to provide expert advice on cancer-related treatments and preventive drugs.

Each committee is composed of representatives from the research science and medical fields. At least one member on every advisory committee must represent the consumer perspective.

Final Approval

As the FDA looks at all the data submitted and the results of its own review, it applies two benchmark questions to each application for drug approval:

- Do the results of well-controlled studies provide substantial evidence of effectiveness?

- Do the results show the product is safe under the conditions of use in the proposed labeling? In this context, "safe" means that potential benefits have been determined to outweigh any risks.

Continued Vigilance

The FDA's responsibility for new drug treatments does not stop with final approval. The Office of Compliance in the Center for Drug Evaluation and Research (CDER) implements and tracks programs to make sure manufacturers comply with current standards and practice regulations. CDER's Office of Drug Marketing, Advertising, and Communication monitors new drug advertising to make sure it is truthful and complete. At the Center for Biologic Evaluation and Research, biologics are followed with the same vigilance after approval. And through a system called MedWatch, the FDA gets feedback from health professionals and consumers on how the new drugs are working, any adverse reactions, and potential problems in labeling and dosage.

Online FDA Resources

The following information from the FDA should help you better understand the drug approval process:

- Center for Drug Evaluation and Research:
  http://www.fda.gov/cder/handbook

- From Test Tube to Patient: New Drug Development in the U.S. – a special January 1995 issue of the magazine FDA Consumer:
  http://www.fda.gov/fdac/special/newdrug/ndd_toc.html

- Milestones in U.S. Food and Drug Law History:
  http://www.fda.gov/opacom/backgrounders/miles.html

- Drug Approvals for Cancer Indications:
  http://www.fda.gov/oashi/cancer/cdrug.html

Getting Drugs to Patients Who Need Them

Clinical trials provide the most important information used by the FDA in determining whether a new drug shows "substantial evidence of effectiveness," or whether an already-approved drug can be used effectively in new ways (for example, to treat or prevent other types of cancer, or at a different dosage). The FDA must certify that a drug has shown promise in laboratory and animal trials before human testing can begin. The trials process includes three main stages and involves continuous review, which ensures that the sponsor can stop the study early if major problems develop or unexpected levels of treatment benefit are found. As with all clinical trials, benefits and risks must be carefully weighed by the researchers conducting the study and the patients who decide to participate.

Not everyone is eligible to participate in a clinical trial. Some patients do not fit the exact requirements for studies, some have rare forms of cancer for which only a limited number of studies are underway, and others are too ill to participate. Working with the NCI and other sponsors, the FDA has established special conditions under which a patient and his or her physician can apply to receive cancer drugs that have not yet been through the approval process. In the past, these special case applications for new drugs were grouped under the name "compassionate uses." More recently, such uses have expanded to include more patients and more categories of investigational drugs.

Access to Investigational Drugs

The process of new drug development has many parts. In the United States, until a drug has been approved by the FDA, it can generally be obtained only through several mechanisms: enrollment in a clinical trial studying the drug, an expanded access program or special exemption/compassionate use programs. For more information about investigational drugs, go to **http://cis.nci.nih.gov/fact/7_46.htm** to view the NCI's fact sheet entitled "Access to Investigational Drugs: Questions and Answers".

"Group C" Drugs

In the 1970s, researchers from the NCI became concerned about the lag between the date when an investigational drug was found to have anti-tumor activity and the time that drug became available on the market. Working with the FDA, the NCI established the "Group C" classification to allow access to drugs with reproducible activity. Group C drugs are provided to properly trained physicians who have registered using a special form to assure that their patient qualifies under guideline protocols for the drug. Each Group C drug protocol specifies patient eligibility, reporting methodology, and drug use. Not only does Group C designation (now called Group C/Treatment INDs) speed new drugs to patients who need them most, but the process also allows the NCI to gather important information on the safety as well as activity of the drugs in the settings in which they will be most used after final FDA approval. Drugs are placed in the Group C category by agreement between the FDA and the NCI. Group C drugs are always provided free of charge, and the Health Care Financing Administration provides coverage for care associated with Group C therapy.

Treatment INDs

In 1987, the FDA began authorizing the use of new drugs still in the development process to treat certain seriously ill patients. In these cases, the process is referred to as a treatment investigational new drug application (Treatment IND). Clinical trials of the new drug must already be underway and have demonstrated positive results that are reproducible. The FDA sets guidelines about what constitutes serious and life-threatening illnesses, how much must already be known about a drug's side effects and benefits, and where physicians can obtain the drug for treatment. For many seriously ill patients, the risks associated with taking a not-yet-completely proven drug are outweighed by the possible benefits.

Accelerated Approval

"Accelerated approval" is the short-hand term for the FDA's new review system which, in the 1990s, has been used to ensure rapid approval while at the same time putting new safeguards into place. Accelerated approval is based on "surrogate endpoint" judgments: FDA can grant marketing approval to drugs and treatments that, according to certain indicators, prove they are likely to have beneficial effects on a disease or condition, even before such direct benefits have been shown clinically. Accelerated approval does NOT mean that additional clinical trials are not needed or that FDA stops gathering information about the effects of the drug; a follow-up study is required to demonstrate activity by more conventional endpoints.

Researching Orphan Drugs

Orphan drugs are a special class of pharmaceuticals used by patients who are unaffected by existing treatments or with illnesses for which no known drug is effective. Orphan drugs are most commonly prescribed or developed for "rare" diseases or conditions.[79] According to the FDA, an orphan drug (or biological) may already be approved, or it may still be experimental. A drug becomes an "orphan" when it receives orphan designation from the Office of Orphan Products Development at the FDA.[80] Orphan designation qualifies the sponsor to receive certain benefits from the U.S. Government in exchange for developing the drug. The drug must then undergo the new drug approval process as any other drug would. To date, over 1000 orphan products have been designated, and over 200 have been approved for marketing. Historically, the approval time for orphan products as a group has been considerably shorter than the approval time for other drugs. This is due to the fact that many orphan products receive expedited review because they are developed for serious or life-threatening diseases.

The cost of orphan products is determined by the sponsor of the drug and can vary greatly. Reimbursement rates for drug expenses are set by each insurance company and outlined in your policy. Insurance companies will generally reimburse for orphan products that have been approved for marketing, but may not reimburse for products that are considered experimental. Consult your insurance company about specific reimbursement policies. If an orphan product has been approved for marketing, it will be available through the normal pharmaceutical supply channels. If the product has not been approved, the sponsor may make the product available on a compassionate-use basis.[81]

---

[79] The U.S. Food and Drug Administration defines a rare disease or condition as "any disease or condition which affects less than 200,000 persons in the United States, or affects more than 200,000 in the United States and for which there is no reasonable expectation that the cost of developing and making available in the United States a drug for such disease or condition will be recovered from sales in the United States of such drug." Adapted from the U.S. Food and Drug Administration: **http://www.fda.gov/opacom/laws/orphandg.htm**.
[80] The following is adapted from the U.S. Food and Drug Administration: **http://www.fda.gov/orphan/faq/index.htm**.
[81] For contact information on sponsors of orphan products, contact the Office of Orphan Products Development (**http://www.fda.gov/orphan/**). General inquiries may be routed to

Although the list of orphan drugs is revised on a daily basis, you can quickly research orphan drugs that might be applicable to adult acute lymphoblastic leukemia using the database managed by the National Organization for Rare Disorders, Inc. (NORD), located at **www.raredisease.org**. Simply go to their general search page and select "Orphan Drug Designation Database." On this page (**http://www.rarediseases.org/search/noddsearch.html**), type "adult acute lymphoblastic leukemia" or a synonym into the search box and click "Submit Query." When you see a list of drugs, understand that not all of the drugs may be relevant. Some may have been withdrawn from orphan status. Write down or print out the name of each drug and the relevant contact information. From there, visit the Pharmacopeia Web site and type the name of each orphan drug into the search box on **http://www.nlm.nih.gov/medlineplus/druginformation.html**. Read about each drug in detail and consult your doctor to find out if you might benefit from these medications. You or your physician may need to contact the sponsor or NORD.

NORD conducts "early access programs for investigational new drugs (IND) under the Food and Drug Administration's (FDA's) approval 'Treatment INDs' programs which allow for a limited number of individuals to receive investigational drugs before FDA marketing approval." If the orphan product about which you are seeking information is approved for marketing, information on side effects can be found on the product's label. If the product is not approved, you or your physician should consult the sponsor.

The following is a list of orphan drugs currently listed in the NORD Orphan Drug Designation Database for adult acute lymphoblastic leukemia or related conditions:

- **clofarabine (trade name: Clofarex)**
  http://www.rarediseases.org/nord/search/nodd_full?code=1240

- **clofarabine (trade name: Clofarex)**
  http://www.rarediseases.org/nord/search/nodd_full?code=1264

- **Technetium Tc-99m murine monoclonal antibody (IgG2 (trade name: LymphoScan)**
  http://www.rarediseases.org/nord/search/nodd_full?code=311

---

the main office: Office of Orphan Products Development (HF-35); Food and Drug Administration, 5600 Fishers Lane, Rockville, MD 20857; Voice: (301) 827-3666 or (800) 300-7469; FAX: (301) 443-4915.

Contraindications and Interactions (Hidden Dangers)

Some of the medications mentioned in the previous discussions can be problematic for patients with adult acute lymphoblastic leukemia--not because they are used in the treatment process, but because of contraindications, or side effects. Medications with contraindications are those that could react with drugs used to treat adult acute lymphoblastic leukemia or potentially create deleterious side effects in patients with adult acute lymphoblastic leukemia. You should ask your physician about any contraindications, especially as these might apply to other medications that you may be taking for common ailments.

Drug-drug interactions occur when two or more drugs react with each other. This drug-drug interaction may cause you to experience an unexpected side effect. Drug interactions may make your medications less effective, cause unexpected side effects, or increase the action of a particular drug. Some drug interactions can even be harmful to you.

Be sure to read the label every time you use a nonprescription or prescription drug, and take the time to learn about drug interactions. These precautions may be critical to your health. You can reduce the risk of potentially harmful drug interactions and side effects with a little bit of knowledge and common sense.

Drug labels contain important information about ingredients, uses, warnings, and directions which you should take the time to read and understand. Labels also include warnings about possible drug interactions. Further, drug labels may change as new information becomes available. This is why it's especially important to read the label every time you use a medication. When your doctor prescribes a new drug, discuss all over-the-counter and prescription medications, dietary supplements, vitamins, botanicals, minerals and herbals you take as well as the foods you eat. Ask your pharmacist for the package insert for each prescription drug you take. The package insert provides more information about potential drug interactions.

A Final Warning

At some point, you may hear of alternative medications from friends, relatives, or in the news media. Advertisements may suggest that certain alternative drugs can produce positive results for patients with adult acute lymphoblastic leukemia. Exercise caution--some of these drugs may have fraudulent claims, and others may actually hurt you. The Food and Drug Administration (FDA) is the official U.S. agency charged with discovering which medications are likely to improve the health of patients with adult acute lymphoblastic leukemia. The FDA warns patients to watch out for[82]:

- Secret formulas (real scientists share what they know)

- Amazing breakthroughs or miracle cures (real breakthroughs don't happen very often; when they do, real scientists do not call them amazing or miracles)

- Quick, painless, or guaranteed cures

- If it sounds too good to be true, it probably isn't true.

If you have any questions about any kind of medical treatment, the FDA may have an office near you. Look for their number in the blue pages of the phone book. You can also contact the FDA through its toll-free number, 1-888-INFO-FDA (1-888-463-6332), or on the World Wide Web at **www.fda.gov**.

General References

In addition to the resources provided earlier in this chapter, the following general references describe medications (sorted alphabetically by title; hyperlinks provide rankings, information and reviews at Amazon.com):

- **Antifolate Drugs in Cancer Therapy (Cancer Drug Discovery and Development)** by Ann L. Jackman (Editor); Hardcover: 480 pages; (March 1999), Humana Press; ISBN: 0896035964; **http://www.amazon.com/exec/obidos/ASIN/0896035964/icongroupinterna**

- **Consumers Guide to Cancer Drugs** by Gail M. Wilkes, et al; Paperback - 448 pages, 1st edition (January 15, 2000), Jones & Bartlett Publishing; ISBN: 0763711705; **http://www.amazon.com/exec/obidos/ASIN/0763711705/icongroupinterna**

- **Patient Education Guide to Oncology Drugs (Book with CD-ROM)** by Gail M. Wilkes, et al; CD-ROM - 447 pages, 1st edition (January 15, 2000), Jones & Bartlett Publishing; ISBN: 076371173X; **http://www.amazon.com/exec/obidos/ASIN/076371173X/icongroupinterna**

---

[82] This section has been adapted from http://www.fda.gov/opacom/lowlit/medfraud.html.

- **The Role of Multiple Intensification in Medical Oncology** by M. S. Aapro (Editor), D. Maraninchi (Editor); Hardcover (June 1998), Springer Verlag; ISBN: 3540635432; http://www.amazon.com/exec/obidos/ASIN/3540635432/icongroupinterna

Vocabulary Builder

The following vocabulary builder provides definitions of words used in this chapter that have not been defined in previous chapters:

Compassionate: A process for providing experimental drugs to very sick patients who have no treatment options. [NIH]

Contraindications: Any factor or sign that it is unwise to pursue a certain kind of action or treatment, e. g. giving a general anesthetic to a person with pneumonia. [NIH]

Therapeutics: The branch of medicine which is concerned with the treatment of diseases, palliative or curative. [NIH]

APPENDIX B. RESEARCHING NUTRITION

Overview

Since the time of Hippocrates, doctors have understood the importance of diet and nutrition to patients' health and well-being. Since then, they have accumulated an impressive archive of studies and knowledge dedicated to this subject. Based on their experience, doctors and healthcare providers may recommend particular dietary supplements to patients with adult acute lymphoblastic leukemia. Any dietary recommendation is based on a patient's age, body mass, gender, lifestyle, eating habits, food preferences, and health condition. It is therefore likely that different patients with adult acute lymphoblastic leukemia may be given different recommendations. Some recommendations may be directly related to adult acute lymphoblastic leukemia, while others may be more related to the patient's general health. These recommendations, themselves, may differ from what official sources recommend for the average person.

In this chapter we will begin by briefly reviewing the essentials of diet and nutrition that will broadly frame more detailed discussions of adult acute lymphoblastic leukemia. We will then show you how to find studies dedicated specifically to nutrition and adult acute lymphoblastic leukemia.

Food and Nutrition: General Principles

What Are Essential Foods?

Food is generally viewed by official sources as consisting of six basic elements: (1) fluids, (2) carbohydrates, (3) protein, (4) fats, (5) vitamins, and

(6) minerals. Consuming a combination of these elements is considered to be a healthy diet:

- **Fluids** are essential to human life as 80-percent of the body is composed of water. Water is lost via urination, sweating, diarrhea, vomiting, diuretics (drugs that increase urination), caffeine, and physical exertion.

- **Carbohydrates** are the main source for human energy (thermoregulation) and the bulk of typical diets. They are mostly classified as being either simple or complex. Simple carbohydrates include sugars which are often consumed in the form of cookies, candies, or cakes. Complex carbohydrates consist of starches and dietary fibers. Starches are consumed in the form of pastas, breads, potatoes, rice, and other foods. Soluble fibers can be eaten in the form of certain vegetables, fruits, oats, and legumes. Insoluble fibers include brown rice, whole grains, certain fruits, wheat bran and legumes.

- **Proteins** are eaten to build and repair human tissues. Some foods that are high in protein are also high in fat and calories. Food sources for protein include nuts, meat, fish, cheese, and other dairy products.

- **Fats** are consumed for both energy and the absorption of certain vitamins. There are many types of fats, with many general publications recommending the intake of unsaturated fats or those low in cholesterol.

Vitamins and minerals are fundamental to human health, growth, and, in some cases, disease prevention. Most are consumed in your diet (exceptions being vitamins K and D which are produced by intestinal bacteria and sunlight on the skin, respectively). Each vitamin and mineral plays a different role in health. The following outlines essential vitamins:

- **Vitamin A** is important to the health of your eyes, hair, bones, and skin; sources of vitamin A include foods such as eggs, carrots, and cantaloupe.

- **Vitamin B^1**, also known as thiamine, is important for your nervous system and energy production; food sources for thiamine include meat, peas, fortified cereals, bread, and whole grains.

- **Vitamin B^2**, also known as riboflavin, is important for your nervous system and muscles, but is also involved in the release of proteins from nutrients; food sources for riboflavin include dairy products, leafy vegetables, meat, and eggs.

- **Vitamin B^3**, also known as niacin, is important for healthy skin and helps the body use energy; food sources for niacin include peas, peanuts, fish, and whole grains

- **Vitamin B^6**, also known as pyridoxine, is important for the regulation of cells in the nervous system and is vital for blood formation; food sources for pyridoxine include bananas, whole grains, meat, and fish.

- **Vitamin B^{12}** is vital for a healthy nervous system and for the growth of red blood cells in bone marrow; food sources for vitamin B^{12} include yeast, milk, fish, eggs, and meat.

- **Vitamin C** allows the body's immune system to fight various diseases, strengthens body tissue, and improves the body's use of iron; food sources for vitamin C include a wide variety of fruits and vegetables.

- **Vitamin D** helps the body absorb calcium which strengthens bones and teeth; food sources for vitamin D include oily fish and dairy products.

- **Vitamin E** can help protect certain organs and tissues from various degenerative diseases; food sources for vitamin E include margarine, vegetables, eggs, and fish.

- **Vitamin K** is essential for bone formation and blood clotting; common food sources for vitamin K include leafy green vegetables.

- **Folic Acid** maintains healthy cells and blood and, when taken by a pregnant woman, can prevent her fetus from developing neural tube defects; food sources for folic acid include nuts, fortified breads, leafy green vegetables, and whole grains.

It should be noted that it is possible to overdose on certain vitamins which become toxic if consumed in excess (e.g. vitamin A, D, E and K).

Like vitamins, minerals are chemicals that are required by the body to remain in good health. Because the human body does not manufacture these chemicals internally, we obtain them from food and other dietary sources. The more important minerals include:

- **Calcium** is needed for healthy bones, teeth, and muscles, but also helps the nervous system function; food sources for calcium include dry beans, peas, eggs, and dairy products.

- **Chromium** is helpful in regulating sugar levels in blood; food sources for chromium include egg yolks, raw sugar, cheese, nuts, beets, whole grains, and meat.

- **Fluoride** is used by the body to help prevent tooth decay and to reinforce bone strength; sources of fluoride include drinking water and certain brands of toothpaste.

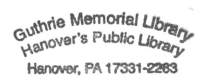

- **Iodine** helps regulate the body's use of energy by synthesizing into the hormone thyroxine; food sources include leafy green vegetables, nuts, egg yolks, and red meat.

- **Iron** helps maintain muscles and the formation of red blood cells and certain proteins; food sources for iron include meat, dairy products, eggs, and leafy green vegetables.

- **Magnesium** is important for the production of DNA, as well as for healthy teeth, bones, muscles, and nerves; food sources for magnesium include dried fruit, dark green vegetables, nuts, and seafood.

- **Phosphorous** is used by the body to work with calcium to form bones and teeth; food sources for phosphorous include eggs, meat, cereals, and dairy products.

- **Selenium** primarily helps maintain normal heart and liver functions; food sources for selenium include wholegrain cereals, fish, meat, and dairy products.

- **Zinc** helps wounds heal, the formation of sperm, and encourage rapid growth and energy; food sources include dried beans, shellfish, eggs, and nuts.

The United States government periodically publishes recommended diets and consumption levels of the various elements of food. Again, your doctor may encourage deviations from the average official recommendation based on your specific condition. To learn more about basic dietary guidelines, visit the Web site: **http://www.health.gov/dietaryguidelines/**. Based on these guidelines, many foods are required to list the nutrition levels on the food's packaging. Labeling Requirements are listed at the following site maintained by the Food and Drug Administration: **http://www.cfsan.fda.gov/~dms/lab-cons.html**. When interpreting these requirements, the government recommends that consumers become familiar with the following abbreviations before reading FDA literature:[83]

- **DVs (Daily Values):** A new dietary reference term that will appear on the food label. It is made up of two sets of references, DRVs and RDIs.

- **DRVs (Daily Reference Values):** A set of dietary references that applies to fat, saturated fat, cholesterol, carbohydrate, protein, fiber, sodium, and potassium.

- **RDIs (Reference Daily Intakes):** A set of dietary references based on the Recommended Dietary Allowances for essential vitamins and minerals

---

[83] Adapted from the FDA: **http://www.fda.gov/fdac/special/foodlabel/dvs.html**.

and, in selected groups, protein. The name "RDI" replaces the term "U.S. RDA."

- **RDAs (Recommended Dietary Allowances):** A set of estimated nutrient allowances established by the National Academy of Sciences. It is updated periodically to reflect current scientific knowledge.

What Are Dietary Supplements?[84]

Dietary supplements are widely available through many commercial sources, including health food stores, grocery stores, pharmacies, and by mail. Dietary supplements are provided in many forms including tablets, capsules, powders, gel-tabs, extracts, and liquids. Historically in the United States, the most prevalent type of dietary supplement was a multivitamin/mineral tablet or capsule that was available in pharmacies, either by prescription or "over the counter." Supplements containing strictly herbal preparations were less widely available. Currently in the United States, a wide array of supplement products are available, including vitamin, mineral, other nutrients, and botanical supplements as well as ingredients and extracts of animal and plant origin.

The Office of Dietary Supplements (ODS) of the National Institutes of Health is the official agency of the United States which has the expressed goal of acquiring "new knowledge to help prevent, detect, diagnose, and treat disease and disability, from the rarest genetic disorder to the common cold."[85] According to the ODS, dietary supplements can have an important impact on the prevention and management of disease and on the maintenance of health.[86] The ODS notes that considerable research on the effects of dietary supplements has been conducted in Asia and Europe where the use of plant products, in particular, has a long tradition. However, the overwhelming majority of supplements have not been studied scientifically.

---

[84] This discussion has been adapted from the NIH: **http://ods.od.nih.gov/showpage.aspx?pageid=46**.

[85] Contact: The Office of Dietary Supplements, National Institutes of Health, Building 31, Room 1B29, 31 Center Drive, MSC 2086, Bethesda, Maryland 20892-2086, Tel: (301) 435-2920, Fax: (301) 480-1845, E-mail: ods@nih.gov.

[86] Adapted from **http://ods.od.nih.gov/showpage.aspx?pageid=2**. The Dietary Supplement Health and Education Act defines dietary supplements as "a product (other than tobacco) intended to supplement the diet that bears or contains one or more of the following dietary ingredients: a vitamin, mineral, amino acid, herb or other botanical; or a dietary substance for use to supplement the diet by increasing the total dietary intake; or a concentrate, metabolite, constituent, extract, or combination of any ingredient described above; and intended for ingestion in the form of a capsule, powder, softgel, or gelcap, and not represented as a conventional food or as a sole item of a meal or the diet."

To explore the role of dietary supplements in the improvement of health care, the ODS plans, organizes, and supports conferences, workshops, and symposia on scientific topics related to dietary supplements. The ODS often works in conjunction with other NIH Institutes and Centers, other government agencies, professional organizations, and public advocacy groups.

To learn more about official information on dietary supplements, visit the ODS site at **http://dietary-supplements.info.nih.gov/**. Or contact:

> **The Office of Dietary Supplements**
> National Institutes of Health
> Building 31, Room 1B29
> 31 Center Drive, MSC 2086
> Bethesda, Maryland 20892-2086
> Tel: (301) 435-2920
> Fax: (301) 480-1845
> E-mail: ods@nih.gov

Finding Studies on Adult Acute Lymphoblastic Leukemia

The NIH maintains an office dedicated to patient nutrition and diet. The National Institutes of Health's Office of Dietary Supplements (ODS) offers a searchable bibliographic database called the IBIDS (International Bibliographic Information on Dietary Supplements). The IBIDS contains over 460,000 scientific citations and summaries about dietary supplements and nutrition as well as references to published international, scientific literature on dietary supplements such as vitamins, minerals, and botanicals.[87] IBIDS is available to the public free of charge through the ODS Internet page: **http://ods.od.nih.gov/databases/ibids.html**.

After entering the search area, you have three choices: (1) IBIDS Consumer Database, (2) Full IBIDS Database, or (3) Peer Reviewed Citations Only. We recommend that you start with the Consumer Database. While you may not find references for the topics that are of most interest to you, check back periodically as this database is frequently updated. More studies can be found by searching the Full IBIDS Database. Healthcare professionals and

---

[87] Adapted from **http://ods.od.nih.gov**. IBIDS is produced by the Office of Dietary Supplements (ODS) at the National Institutes of Health to assist the public, healthcare providers, educators, and researchers in locating credible, scientific information on dietary supplements. IBIDS was developed and will be maintained through an interagency partnership with the Food and Nutrition Information Center of the National Agricultural Library, U.S. Department of Agriculture.

researchers generally use the third option, which lists peer-reviewed citations. In all cases, we suggest that you take advantage of the "Advanced Search" option that allows you to retrieve up to 100 fully explained references in a comprehensive format. Type "adult acute lymphoblastic leukemia" (or synonyms) into the search box. To narrow the search, you can also select the "Title" field.

The following information is typical of that found when using the "Full IBIDS Database" when searching using "adult acute lymphoblastic leukemia" (or a synonym):

- **Age-adapted induction treatment of acute lymphoblastic leukemia in the elderly and assessment of maintenance with interferon combined with chemotherapy. A multicentric prospective study in forty patients. French Group for Treatment of Adult Acute Lymphoblastic Leukemia.**
  Author(s): Delannoy, A : Sebban, C : Cony Makhoul, P : Cazin, B : Cordonnier, C : Bouabdallah, R : Cahn, J Y : Dreyfus, F : Sadoun, A : Vernant, J P : Gay, C : Broustet, A : Michaux, J L : Fiere, D
  Source: Leukemia.

- **Allogeneic bone marrow transplantation in adult acute lymphoblastic leukemia in first complete remission: a comparative study. French Group of Therapy of Adult Acute Lymphoblastic Leukemia.**
  Author(s): Sebban, C : Lepage, E : Vernant, J P : Gluckman, E : Attal, M : Reiffers, J : Sutton, L : Racadot, E : Michallet, M : Maraninchi, D : et al.
  Source: J-Clin-Oncol.

- **Cytarabine with high-dose mitoxantrone induces rapid complete remissions in adult acute lymphoblastic leukemia without the use of vincristine or prednisone.**
  Author(s): Weiss, M : Maslak, P : Feldman, E : Berman, E : Bertino, J : Gee, T : Megherian, L : Seiter, K : Scheinberg, D : Golde, D
  Source: J-Clin-Oncol.

- **Daunorubicin continuous infusion induces more toxicity than bolus infusion in acute lymphoblastic leukemia induction regimen: a randomized study.**
  Author(s): Hunault Berger, M : Milpied, N : Bernard, M : Jouet, J P : Delain, M : Desablens, B : Sadoun, A : Guilhot, F : Casassus, P : Ifrah, N
  Source: Leukemia.

- **Estimated 6-year event-free survival of 55% in 60 consecutive adult acute lymphoblastic leukemia patients treated with an intensive phase II protocol based on high induction dose of daunorubicin.**
  Author(s): Todeschini, G : Tecchio, C : Meneghini, V : Pizzolo, G : Veneri, D : Zanotti, R : Ricetti, M M : Solero, P : April, F : Perona, G

Source: Leukemia.

- **High efficacy of the German multicenter ALL (GMALL) protocol for treatment of adult acute lymphoblastic leukemia (ALL)--a single-institution study.**
  Author(s): Scherrer, R : Bettelheim, P : Geissler, K : Jager, U : Knobl, P : Kyrle, P A : Laczika, K : Mitterbauer, G : Neumann, E : Schneider, B : et al.
  Source: Ann-Hematol.

- **In vitro culture with prednisolone increases BCL-2 protein expression in adult acute lymphoblastic leukemia cells.**
  Author(s): Tosi, P : Visani, G : Ottaviani, E : Manfroi, S : Tura, S
  Source: Am-J-Hematol.

- **Persistence of peripheral blood and bone marrow blasts during remission induction in adult acute lymphoblastic leukemia confers a poor prognosis depending on treatment intensity.**
  Author(s): Cortes, J : Fayad, L : O'Brien, S : Keating, M : Kantarjian, H
  Source: Clin-Cancer-Res.

- **Short-term intensive treatment (V.A.A.P.) of adult acute lymphoblastic leukemia and lymphoblastic lymphoma.**
  Author(s): Willemze, R : Peters, W G : Colly, L P
  Source: Eur-J-Haematol.

- **Successful treatment of adult acute lymphoblastic leukemia after relapse with prednisone, intermediate-dose cytarabine, mitoxantrone, and etoposide (PAME) chemotherapy.**
  Author(s): Milpied, N : Gisselbrecht, C : Harousseau, J L : Sebban, C : Witz, F : Troussard, X : Gratecos, N : Michallet, M : LeBlond, V : Auzanneau, G : et al.
  Source: Cancer.

Federal Resources on Nutrition

In addition to the IBIDS, the United States Department of Health and Human Services (HHS) and the United States Department of Agriculture (USDA) provide many sources of information on general nutrition and health. Recommended resources include:

- healthfinder®, HHS's gateway to health information, including diet and nutrition:
  http://www.healthfinder.gov/scripts/SearchContext.asp?topic=238&page=0

- The United States Department of Agriculture's Web site dedicated to nutrition information: **www.nutrition.gov**

- The Food and Drug Administration's Web site for federal food safety information: **www.foodsafety.gov**

- The National Action Plan on Overweight and Obesity sponsored by the United States Surgeon General: **http://www.surgeongeneral.gov/topics/obesity/**

- The Center for Food Safety and Applied Nutrition has an Internet site sponsored by the Food and Drug Administration and the Department of Health and Human Services: **http://vm.cfsan.fda.gov/**

- Center for Nutrition Policy and Promotion sponsored by the United States Department of Agriculture: **http://www.usda.gov/cnpp/**

- Food and Nutrition Information Center, National Agricultural Library sponsored by the United States Department of Agriculture: **http://www.nal.usda.gov/fnic/**

- Food and Nutrition Service sponsored by the United States Department of Agriculture: **http://www.fns.usda.gov/fns/**

Additional Web Resources

A number of additional Web sites offer encyclopedic information covering food and nutrition. The following is a representative sample:

- AOL: **http://search.aol.com/cat.adp?id=174&layer=&from=subcats**

- Family Village: **http://www.familyvillage.wisc.edu/med_nutrition.html**

- Google: **http://directory.google.com/Top/Health/Nutrition/**

- Open Directory Project: **http://dmoz.org/Health/Nutrition/**

- Yahoo.com: **http://dir.yahoo.com/Health/Nutrition/**

- WebMD®Health: **http://my.webmd.com/nutrition**

- WholeHealthMD.com: **http://www.wholehealthmd.com/reflib/0,1529,,00.html**

Vocabulary Builder

The following vocabulary builder provides definitions of words used in this chapter that have not been defined in previous chapters:

Nerve: A cordlike structure of nervous tissue that connects parts of the nervous system with other tissues of the body and conveys nervous impulses to, or away from, these tissues. [NIH]

Potassium: It is essential to the ability of muscle cells to contract. [NIH]

Sperm: The fecundating fluid of the male. [NIH]

Appendix C. Finding Medical Libraries

Overview

At a medical library you can find medical texts and reference books, consumer health publications, specialty newspapers and magazines, as well as medical journals. In this Appendix, we show you how to quickly find a medical library in your area.

Preparation

Before going to the library, highlight the references mentioned in this sourcebook that you find interesting. Focus on those items that are not available via the Internet, and ask the reference librarian for help with your search. He or she may know of additional resources that could be helpful to you. Most importantly, your local public library and medical libraries have Interlibrary Loan programs with the National Library of Medicine (NLM), one of the largest medical collections in the world. According to the NLM, most of the literature in the general and historical collections of the National Library of Medicine is available on interlibrary loan to any library. NLM's interlibrary loan services are only available to libraries. If you would like to access NLM medical literature, then visit a library in your area that can request the publications for you.[88]

---

[88] Adapted from the NLM: **http://www.nlm.nih.gov/psd/cas/interlibrary.html**.

Finding a Local Medical Library

The quickest method to locate medical libraries is to use the Internet-based directory published by the National Network of Libraries of Medicine (NN/LM). This network includes 4626 members and affiliates that provide many services to librarians, health professionals, and the public. To find a library in your area, simply visit **http://nnlm.gov/members/adv.html** or call 1-800-338-7657.

Medical Libraries in the U.S. and Canada

In addition to the NN/LM, the National Library of Medicine (NLM) lists a number of libraries with reference facilities that are open to the public. The following is the NLM's list and includes hyperlinks to each library's Web site. These Web pages can provide information on hours of operation and other restrictions. The list below is a small sample of libraries recommended by the National Library of Medicine (sorted alphabetically by name of the U.S. state or Canadian province where the library is located)[89]:

- **Alabama:** Health InfoNet of Jefferson County (Jefferson County Library Cooperative, Lister Hill Library of the Health Sciences), **http://www.uab.edu/infonet/**

- **Alabama:** Richard M. Scrushy Library (American Sports Medicine Institute)

- **Arizona:** Samaritan Regional Medical Center: The Learning Center (Samaritan Health System, Phoenix, Arizona), **http://www.samaritan.edu/library/bannerlibs.htm**

- **California:** Kris Kelly Health Information Center (St. Joseph Health System, Humboldt), **http://www.humboldt1.com/~kkhic/index.html**

- **California:** Community Health Library of Los Gatos, **http://www.healthlib.org/orgresources.html**

- **California:** Consumer Health Program and Services (CHIPS) (County of Los Angeles Public Library, Los Angeles County Harbor-UCLA Medical Center Library) - Carson, CA, **http://www.colapublib.org/services/chips.html**

- **California:** Gateway Health Library (Sutter Gould Medical Foundation)

- **California:** Health Library (Stanford University Medical Center), **http://www-med.stanford.edu/healthlibrary/**

---

[89] Abstracted from **http://www.nlm.nih.gov/medlineplus/libraries.html**.

- **California:** Patient Education Resource Center - Health Information and Resources (University of California, San Francisco), **http://sfghdean.ucsf.edu/barnett/PERC/default.asp**
- **California:** Redwood Health Library (Petaluma Health Care District), **http://www.phcd.org/rdwdlib.html**
- **California:** Los Gatos PlaneTree Health Library, **http://planetreesanjose.org/**
- **California:** Sutter Resource Library (Sutter Hospitals Foundation, Sacramento), **http://suttermedicalcenter.org/library/**
- **California:** Health Sciences Libraries (University of California, Davis), **http://www.lib.ucdavis.edu/healthsci/**
- **California:** ValleyCare Health Library & Ryan Comer Cancer Resource Center (ValleyCare Health System, Pleasanton), **http://gaelnet.stmarys-ca.edu/other.libs/gbal/east/vchl.html**
- **California:** Washington Community Health Resource Library (Fremont), **http://www.healthlibrary.org/**
- **Colorado:** William V. Gervasini Memorial Library (Exempla Healthcare), **http://www.saintjosephdenver.org/yourhealth/libraries/**
- **Connecticut:** Hartford Hospital Health Science Libraries (Hartford Hospital), **http://www.harthosp.org/library/**
- **Connecticut:** Healthnet: Connecticut Consumer Health Information Center (University of Connecticut Health Center, Lyman Maynard Stowe Library), **http://library.uchc.edu/departm/hnet/**
- **Connecticut:** Waterbury Hospital Health Center Library (Waterbury Hospital, Waterbury), **http://www.waterburyhospital.com/library/consumer.shtml**
- **Delaware:** Consumer Health Library (Christiana Care Health System, Eugene du Pont Preventive Medicine & Rehabilitation Institute, Wilmington), **http://www.christianacare.org/health_guide/health_guide_pmri_health _info.cfm**
- **Delaware:** Lewis B. Flinn Library (Delaware Academy of Medicine, Wilmington), **http://www.delamed.org/chls.html**
- **Georgia:** Family Resource Library (Medical College of Georgia, Augusta), **http://cmc.mcg.edu/kids_families/fam_resources/fam_res_lib/frl.htm**
- **Georgia:** Health Resource Center (Medical Center of Central Georgia, Macon), **http://www.mccg.org/hrc/hrchome.asp**

- **Hawaii:** Hawaii Medical Library: Consumer Health Information Service (Hawaii Medical Library, Honolulu), **http://hml.org/CHIS/**

- **Idaho:** DeArmond Consumer Health Library (Kootenai Medical Center, Coeur d'Alene), **http://www.nicon.org/DeArmond/index.htm**

- **Illinois:** Health Learning Center of Northwestern Memorial Hospital (Chicago), **http://www.nmh.org/health_info/hlc.html**

- **Illinois:** Medical Library (OSF Saint Francis Medical Center, Peoria), **http://www.osfsaintfrancis.org/general/library/**

- **Kentucky:** Medical Library - Services for Patients, Families, Students & the Public (Central Baptist Hospital, Lexington), **http://www.centralbap.com/education/community/library.cfm**

- **Kentucky:** University of Kentucky - Health Information Library (Chandler Medical Center, Lexington), **http://www.mc.uky.edu/PatientEd/**

- **Louisiana:** Alton Ochsner Medical Foundation Library (Alton Ochsner Medical Foundation, New Orleans), **http://www.ochsner.org/library/**

- **Louisiana:** Louisiana State University Health Sciences Center Medical Library-Shreveport, **http://lib-sh.lsuhsc.edu/**

- **Maine:** Franklin Memorial Hospital Medical Library (Franklin Memorial Hospital, Farmington), **http://www.fchn.org/fmh/lib.htm**

- **Maine:** Gerrish-True Health Sciences Library (Central Maine Medical Center, Lewiston), **http://www.cmmc.org/library/library.html**

- **Maine:** Hadley Parrot Health Science Library (Eastern Maine Healthcare, Bangor), **http://www.emh.org/hll/hpl/guide.htm**

- **Maine:** Maine Medical Center Library (Maine Medical Center, Portland), **http://www.mmc.org/library/**

- **Maine:** Parkview Hospital (Brunswick), **http://www.parkviewhospital.org/**

- **Maine:** Southern Maine Medical Center Health Sciences Library (Southern Maine Medical Center, Biddeford), **http://www.smmc.org/services/service.php3?choice=10**

- **Maine:** Stephens Memorial Hospital's Health Information Library (Western Maine Health, Norway), **http://www.wmhcc.org/Library/**

- **Manitoba, Canada:** Consumer & Patient Health Information Service (University of Manitoba Libraries), **http://www.umanitoba.ca/libraries/units/health/reference/chis.html**

- **Manitoba, Canada:** J.W. Crane Memorial Library (Deer Lodge Centre, Winnipeg), **http://www.deerlodge.mb.ca/crane_library/about.asp**

- **Maryland:** Health Information Center at the Wheaton Regional Library (Montgomery County, Dept. of Public Libraries, Wheaton Regional Library), **http://www.mont.lib.md.us/healthinfo/hic.asp**

- **Massachusetts:** Baystate Medical Center Library (Baystate Health System), **http://www.baystatehealth.com/1024/**

- **Massachusetts:** Boston University Medical Center Alumni Medical Library (Boston University Medical Center), **http://med-libwww.bu.edu/library/lib.html**

- **Massachusetts:** Lowell General Hospital Health Sciences Library (Lowell General Hospital, Lowell), **http://www.lowellgeneral.org/library/HomePageLinks/WWW.htm**

- **Massachusetts:** Paul E. Woodard Health Sciences Library (New England Baptist Hospital, Boston), **http://www.nebh.org/health_lib.asp**

- **Massachusetts:** St. Luke's Hospital Health Sciences Library (St. Luke's Hospital, Southcoast Health System, New Bedford), **http://www.southcoast.org/library/**

- **Massachusetts:** Treadwell Library Consumer Health Reference Center (Massachusetts General Hospital), **http://www.mgh.harvard.edu/library/chrcindex.html**

- **Massachusetts:** UMass HealthNet (University of Massachusetts Medical School, Worcester), **http://healthnet.umassmed.edu/**

- **Michigan:** Botsford General Hospital Library - Consumer Health (Botsford General Hospital, Library & Internet Services), **http://www.botsfordlibrary.org/consumer.htm**

- **Michigan:** Helen DeRoy Medical Library (Providence Hospital and Medical Centers), **http://www.providence-hospital.org/library/**

- **Michigan:** Marquette General Hospital - Consumer Health Library (Marquette General Hospital, Health Information Center), **http://www.mgh.org/center.html**

- **Michigan:** Patient Education Resouce Center - University of Michigan Cancer Center (University of Michigan Comprehensive Cancer Center, Ann Arbor), **http://www.cancer.med.umich.edu/learn/leares.htm**

- **Michigan:** Sladen Library & Center for Health Information Resources - Consumer Health Information (Detroit), **http://www.henryford.com/body.cfm?id=39330**

- **Montana:** Center for Health Information (St. Patrick Hospital and Health Sciences Center, Missoula)

- **National:** Consumer Health Library Directory (Medical Library Association, Consumer and Patient Health Information Section), http://caphis.mlanet.org/directory/index.html

- **National:** National Network of Libraries of Medicine (National Library of Medicine) - provides library services for health professionals in the United States who do not have access to a medical library, http://nnlm.gov/

- **National:** NN/LM List of Libraries Serving the Public (National Network of Libraries of Medicine), http://nnlm.gov/members/

- **Nevada:** Health Science Library, West Charleston Library (Las Vegas-Clark County Library District, Las Vegas), http://www.lvccld.org/special_collections/medical/index.htm

- **New Hampshire:** Dartmouth Biomedical Libraries (Dartmouth College Library, Hanover), http://www.dartmouth.edu/~biomed/resources.htmld/conshealth.htmld

- **New Jersey:** Consumer Health Library (Rahway Hospital, Rahway), http://www.rahwayhospital.com/library.htm

- **New Jersey:** Dr. Walter Phillips Health Sciences Library (Englewood Hospital and Medical Center, Englewood), http://www.englewoodhospital.com/links/index.htm

- **New Jersey:** Meland Foundation (Englewood Hospital and Medical Center, Englewood), http://www.geocities.com/ResearchTriangle/9360/

- **New York:** Choices in Health Information (New York Public Library) - NLM Consumer Pilot Project participant, http://www.nypl.org/branch/health/links.html

- **New York:** Health Information Center (Upstate Medical University, State University of New York, Syracuse), http://www.upstate.edu/library/hic/

- **New York:** Health Sciences Library (Long Island Jewish Medical Center, New Hyde Park), http://www.lij.edu/library/library.html

- **New York:** ViaHealth Medical Library (Rochester General Hospital), http://www.nyam.org/library/

- **Ohio:** Consumer Health Library (Akron General Medical Center, Medical & Consumer Health Library), http://www.akrongeneral.org/hwlibrary.htm

- **Oklahoma:** The Health Information Center at Saint Francis Hospital (Saint Francis Health System, Tulsa), **http://www.sfh-tulsa.com/services/healthinfo.asp**

- **Oregon:** Planetree Health Resource Center (Mid-Columbia Medical Center, The Dalles), **http://www.mcmc.net/phrc/**

- **Pennsylvania:** Community Health Information Library (Milton S. Hershey Medical Center, Hershey), **http://www.hmc.psu.edu/commhealth/**

- **Pennsylvania:** Community Health Resource Library (Geisinger Medical Center, Danville), **http://www.geisinger.edu/education/commlib.shtml**

- **Pennsylvania:** HealthInfo Library (Moses Taylor Hospital, Scranton), **http://www.mth.org/healthwellness.html**

- **Pennsylvania:** Hopwood Library (University of Pittsburgh, Health Sciences Library System, Pittsburgh), **http://www.hsls.pitt.edu/guides/chi/hopwood/index_html**

- **Pennsylvania:** Koop Community Health Information Center (College of Physicians of Philadelphia), **http://www.collphyphil.org/kooppg1.shtml**

- **Pennsylvania:** Learning Resources Center - Medical Library (Susquehanna Health System, Williamsport), **http://www.shscares.org/services/lrc/index.asp**

- **Pennsylvania:** Medical Library (UPMC Health System, Pittsburgh), **http://www.upmc.edu/passavant/library.htm**

- **Quebec, Canada:** Medical Library (Montreal General Hospital), **http://www.mghlib.mcgill.ca/**

- **South Dakota:** Rapid City Regional Hospital Medical Library (Rapid City Regional Hospital), **http://www.rcrh.org/Services/Library/Default.asp**

- **Texas:** Houston HealthWays (Houston Academy of Medicine-Texas Medical Center Library), **http://hhw.library.tmc.edu/**

- **Washington:** Community Health Library (Kittitas Valley Community Hospital), **http://www.kvch.com/**

- **Washington:** Southwest Washington Medical Center Library (Southwest Washington Medical Center, Vancouver), **http://www.swmedicalcenter.com/body.cfm?id=72**

APPENDIX D. YOUR RIGHTS AND INSURANCE

Overview

Any patient with adult acute lymphoblastic leukemia faces a series of issues related more to the healthcare industry than to the medical condition itself. This appendix covers two important topics in this regard: your rights and responsibilities as a patient, and how to get the most out of your medical insurance plan.

Your Rights as a Patient

The President's Advisory Commission on Consumer Protection and Quality in the Healthcare Industry has created the following summary of your rights as a patient.[90]

Information Disclosure

Consumers have the right to receive accurate, easily understood information. Some consumers require assistance in making informed decisions about health plans, health professionals, and healthcare facilities. Such information includes:

- *Health plans.* Covered benefits, cost-sharing, and procedures for resolving complaints, licensure, certification, and accreditation status, comparable measures of quality and consumer satisfaction, provider

---

[90]Adapted from Consumer Bill of Rights and Responsibilities:
http://www.hcqualitycommission.gov/press/cbor.html#head1.

network composition, the procedures that govern access to specialists and emergency services, and care management information.

- *Health professionals.* Education, board certification, and recertification, years of practice, experience performing certain procedures, and comparable measures of quality and consumer satisfaction.

- *Healthcare facilities.* Experience in performing certain procedures and services, accreditation status, comparable measures of quality, worker, and consumer satisfaction, and procedures for resolving complaints.

- *Consumer assistance programs.* Programs must be carefully structured to promote consumer confidence and to work cooperatively with health plans, providers, payers, and regulators. Desirable characteristics of such programs are sponsorship that ensures accountability to the interests of consumers and stable, adequate funding.

Choice of Providers and Plans

Consumers have the right to a choice of healthcare providers that is sufficient to ensure access to appropriate high-quality healthcare. To ensure such choice, the Commission recommends the following:

- *Provider network adequacy.* All health plan networks should provide access to sufficient numbers and types of providers to assure that all covered services will be accessible without unreasonable delay -- including access to emergency services 24 hours a day and 7 days a week. If a health plan has an insufficient number or type of providers to provide a covered benefit with the appropriate degree of specialization, the plan should ensure that the consumer obtains the benefit outside the network at no greater cost than if the benefit were obtained from participating providers.

- *Women's health services.* Women should be able to choose a qualified provider offered by a plan -- such as gynecologists, certified nurse midwives, and other qualified healthcare providers -- for the provision of covered care necessary to provide routine and preventative women's healthcare services.

- *Access to specialists.* Consumers with complex or serious medical conditions who require frequent specialty care should have direct access to a qualified specialist of their choice within a plan's network of providers. Authorizations, when required, should be for an adequate number of direct access visits under an approved treatment plan.

- *Transitional care.* Consumers who are undergoing a course of treatment for a chronic or disabling condition (or who are in the second or third trimester of a pregnancy) at the time they involuntarily change health plans or at a time when a provider is terminated by a plan for other than cause should be able to continue seeing their current specialty providers for up to 90 days (or through completion of postpartum care) to allow for transition of care.

- *Choice of health plans.* Public and private group purchasers should, wherever feasible, offer consumers a choice of high-quality health insurance plans.

Access to Emergency Services

Consumers have the right to access emergency healthcare services when and where the need arises. Health plans should provide payment when a consumer presents to an emergency department with acute symptoms of sufficient severity--including severe pain--such that a "prudent layperson" could reasonably expect the absence of medical attention to result in placing that consumer's health in serious jeopardy, serious impairment to bodily functions, or serious dysfunction of any bodily organ or part.

Participation in Treatment Decisions

Consumers have the right and responsibility to fully participate in all decisions related to their healthcare. Consumers who are unable to fully participate in treatment decisions have the right to be represented by parents, guardians, family members, or other conservators. Physicians and other health professionals should:

- Provide patients with sufficient information and opportunity to decide among treatment options consistent with the informed consent process.

- Discuss all treatment options with a patient in a culturally competent manner, including the option of no treatment at all.

- Ensure that persons with disabilities have effective communications with members of the health system in making such decisions.

- Discuss all current treatments a consumer may be undergoing.

- Discuss all risks, benefits, and consequences to treatment or nontreatment.

- Give patients the opportunity to refuse treatment and to express preferences about future treatment decisions.

- Discuss the use of advance directives -- both living wills and durable powers of attorney for healthcare -- with patients and their designated family members.

- Abide by the decisions made by their patients and/or their designated representatives consistent with the informed consent process.

Health plans, health providers, and healthcare facilities should:

- Disclose to consumers factors -- such as methods of compensation, ownership of or interest in healthcare facilities, or matters of conscience -- that could influence advice or treatment decisions.

- Assure that provider contracts do not contain any so-called "gag clauses" or other contractual mechanisms that restrict healthcare providers' ability to communicate with and advise patients about medically necessary treatment options.

- Be prohibited from penalizing or seeking retribution against healthcare professionals or other health workers for advocating on behalf of their patients.

Respect and Nondiscrimination

Consumers have the right to considerate, respectful care from all members of the healthcare industry at all times and under all circumstances. An environment of mutual respect is essential to maintain a quality healthcare system. To assure that right, the Commission recommends the following:

- Consumers must not be discriminated against in the delivery of healthcare services consistent with the benefits covered in their policy, or as required by law, based on race, ethnicity, national origin, religion, sex, age, mental or physical disability, sexual orientation, genetic information, or source of payment.

- Consumers eligible for coverage under the terms and conditions of a health plan or program, or as required by law, must not be discriminated against in marketing and enrollment practices based on race, ethnicity, national origin, religion, sex, age, mental or physical disability, sexual orientation, genetic information, or source of payment.

Confidentiality of Health Information

Consumers have the right to communicate with healthcare providers in confidence and to have the confidentiality of their individually identifiable healthcare information protected. Consumers also have the right to review and copy their own medical records and request amendments to their records.

Complaints and Appeals

Consumers have the right to a fair and efficient process for resolving differences with their health plans, healthcare providers, and the institutions that serve them, including a rigorous system of internal review and an independent system of external review. A free copy of the Patient's Bill of Rights is available from the American Hospital Association.[91]

Patient Responsibilities

Treatment is a two-way street between you and your healthcare providers. To underscore the importance of finance in modern healthcare as well as your responsibility for the financial aspects of your care, the President's Advisory Commission on Consumer Protection and Quality in the Healthcare Industry has proposed that patients understand the following "Consumer Responsibilities."[92] In a healthcare system that protects consumers' rights, it is reasonable to expect and encourage consumers to assume certain responsibilities. Greater individual involvement by the consumer in his or her care increases the likelihood of achieving the best outcome and helps support a quality-oriented, cost-conscious environment. Such responsibilities include:

- Take responsibility for maximizing healthy habits such as exercising, not smoking, and eating a healthy diet.

- Work collaboratively with healthcare providers in developing and carrying out agreed-upon treatment plans.

- Disclose relevant information and clearly communicate wants and needs.

---

[91] To order your free copy of the Patient's Bill of Rights, telephone 312-422-3000 or visit the American Hospital Association's Web site: http://www.aha.org. Click on "Resource Center," go to "Search" at bottom of page, and then type in "Patient's Bill of Rights." The Patient's Bill of Rights is also available from Fax on Demand, at 312-422-2020, document number 471124.

[92] Adapted from http://www.hcqualitycommission.gov/press/cbor.html#head1.

- Use your health insurance plan's internal complaint and appeal processes to address your concerns.

- Avoid knowingly spreading disease.

- Recognize the reality of risks, the limits of the medical science, and the human fallibility of the healthcare professional.

- Be aware of a healthcare provider's obligation to be reasonably efficient and equitable in providing care to other patients and the community.

- Become knowledgeable about your health plan's coverage and options (when available) including all covered benefits, limitations, and exclusions, rules regarding use of network providers, coverage and referral rules, appropriate processes to secure additional information, and the process to appeal coverage decisions.

- Show respect for other patients and health workers.

- Make a good-faith effort to meet financial obligations.

- Abide by administrative and operational procedures of health plans, healthcare providers, and Government health benefit programs.

Choosing an Insurance Plan

There are a number of official government agencies that help consumers understand their healthcare insurance choices.[93] The U.S. Department of Labor, in particular, recommends ten ways to make your health benefits choices work best for you.[94]

1. Your options are important. There are many different types of health benefit plans. Find out which one your employer offers, then check out the plan, or plans, offered. Your employer's human resource office, the health plan administrator, or your union can provide information to help you match your needs and preferences with the available plans. The more information you have, the better your healthcare decisions will be.

2. Reviewing the benefits available. Do the plans offered cover preventive care, well-baby care, vision or dental care? Are there deductibles? Answers to these questions can help determine the out-of-pocket expenses you may face. Matching your needs and those of your family members will result in

---

[93] More information about quality across programs is provided at the following AHRQ Web site: **http://www.ahrq.gov/consumer/qntascii/qnthplan.htm**.
[94] Adapted from the Department of Labor:
http://www.dol.gov/dol/pwba/public/pubs/health/top10-text.html.

the best possible benefits. Cheapest may not always be best. Your goal is high quality health benefits.

3. Look for quality. The quality of healthcare services varies, but quality can be measured. You should consider the quality of healthcare in deciding among the healthcare plans or options available to you. Not all health plans, doctors, hospitals and other providers give the highest quality care. Fortunately, there is quality information you can use right now to help you compare your healthcare choices. Find out how you can measure quality. Consult the U.S. Department of Health and Human Services publication "Your Guide to Choosing Quality Health Care" on the Internet at **www.ahcpr.gov/consumer**.

4. Your plan's summary plan description (SPD) provides a wealth of information. Your health plan administrator can provide you with a copy of your plan's SPD. It outlines your benefits and your legal rights under the Employee Retirement Income Security Act (ERISA), the federal law that protects your health benefits. It should contain information about the coverage of dependents, what services will require a co-pay, and the circumstances under which your employer can change or terminate a health benefits plan. Save the SPD and all other health plan brochures and documents, along with memos or correspondence from your employer relating to health benefits.

5. Assess your benefit coverage as your family status changes. Marriage, divorce, childbirth or adoption, and the death of a spouse are all life events that may signal a need to change your health benefits. You, your spouse and dependent children may be eligible for a special enrollment period under provisions of the Health Insurance Portability and Accountability Act (HIPAA). Even without life-changing events, the information provided by your employer should tell you how you can change benefits or switch plans, if more than one plan is offered. If your spouse's employer also offers a health benefits package, consider coordinating both plans for maximum coverage.

6. Changing jobs and other life events can affect your health benefits. Under the Consolidated Omnibus Budget Reconciliation Act (COBRA), you, your covered spouse, and your dependent children may be eligible to purchase extended health coverage under your employer's plan if you lose your job, change employers, get divorced, or upon occurrence of certain other events. Coverage can range from 18 to 36 months depending on your situation. COBRA applies to most employers with 20 or more workers and requires your plan to notify you of your rights. Most plans require eligible individuals to make their COBRA election within 60 days of the plan's notice. Be sure to follow up with your plan sponsor if you don't receive notice, and make sure you respond within the allotted time.

7. HIPAA can also help if you are changing jobs, particularly if you have a medical condition. HIPAA generally limits pre-existing condition exclusions to a maximum of 12 months (18 months for late enrollees). HIPAA also requires this maximum period to be reduced by the length of time you had prior "creditable coverage." You should receive a certificate documenting your prior creditable coverage from your old plan when coverage ends.

8. Plan for retirement. Before you retire, find out what health benefits, if any, extend to you and your spouse during your retirement years. Consult with your employer's human resources office, your union, the plan administrator, and check your SPD. Make sure there is no conflicting information among these sources about the benefits you will receive or the circumstances under which they can change or be eliminated. With this information in hand, you can make other important choices, like finding out if you are eligible for Medicare and Medigap insurance coverage.

9. Know how to file an appeal if your health benefits claim is denied. Understand how your plan handles grievances and where to make appeals of the plan's decisions. Keep records and copies of correspondence. Check your health benefits package and your SPD to determine who is responsible for handling problems with benefit claims. Contact PWBA for customer service assistance if you are unable to obtain a response to your complaint.

10. You can take steps to improve the quality of the healthcare and the health benefits you receive. Look for and use things like Quality Reports and Accreditation Reports whenever you can. Quality reports may contain consumer ratings -- how satisfied consumers are with the doctors in their plan, for instance-- and clinical performance measures -- how well a healthcare organization prevents and treats illness. Accreditation reports provide information on how accredited organizations meet national standards, and often include clinical performance measures. Look for these quality measures whenever possible. Consult "Your Guide to Choosing Quality Health Care" on the Internet at **www.ahcpr.gov/consumer**.

Medicare and Medicaid

Illness strikes both rich and poor families. For low-income families, Medicaid is available to defer the costs of treatment. The Health Care Financing

Administration (HCFA) administers Medicare, the nation's largest health insurance program, which covers 39 million Americans. In the following pages, you will learn the basics about Medicare insurance as well as useful contact information on how to find more in-depth information about Medicaid.[95]

Who Is Eligible for Medicare?

Generally, you are eligible for Medicare if you or your spouse worked for at least 10 years in Medicare-covered employment and you are 65 years old and a citizen or permanent resident of the United States. You might also qualify for coverage if you are under age 65 but have a disability or End-Stage Renal disease (permanent kidney failure requiring dialysis or transplant). Here are some simple guidelines:

You can get Part A at age 65 without having to pay premiums if:

- You are already receiving retirement benefits from Social Security or the Railroad Retirement Board.

- You are eligible to receive Social Security or Railroad benefits but have not yet filed for them.

- You or your spouse had Medicare-covered government employment.

If you are under 65, you can get Part A without having to pay premiums if:

- You have received Social Security or Railroad Retirement Board disability benefit for 24 months.

- You are a kidney dialysis or kidney transplant patient.

Medicare has two parts:

- Part A (Hospital Insurance). Most people do not have to pay for Part A.
- Part B (Medical Insurance). Most people pay monthly for Part B.

---

[95] This section has been adapted from the Official U.S. Site for Medicare Information: **http://www.medicare.gov/Basics/Overview.asp**.

Part A (Hospital Insurance)

Helps Pay For: Inpatient hospital care, care in critical access hospitals (small facilities that give limited outpatient and inpatient services to people in rural areas) and skilled nursing facilities, hospice care, and some home healthcare.

Cost: Most people get Part A automatically when they turn age 65. You do not have to pay a monthly payment called a premium for Part A because you or a spouse paid Medicare taxes while you were working.

If you (or your spouse) did not pay Medicare taxes while you were working and you are age 65 or older, you still may be able to buy Part A. If you are not sure you have Part A, look on your red, white, and blue Medicare card. It will show "Hospital Part A" on the lower left corner of the card. You can also call the Social Security Administration toll free at 1-800-772-1213 or call your local Social Security office for more information about buying Part A. If you get benefits from the Railroad Retirement Board, call your local RRB office or 1-800-808-0772. For more information, call your Fiscal Intermediary about Part A bills and services. The phone number for the Fiscal Intermediary office in your area can be obtained from the following Web site: **http://www.medicare.gov/Contacts/home.asp**.

Part B (Medical Insurance)

Helps Pay For: Doctors, services, outpatient hospital care, and some other medical services that Part A does not cover, such as the services of physical and occupational therapists, and some home healthcare. Part B helps pay for covered services and supplies when they are medically necessary.

Cost: As of 2001, you pay the Medicare Part B premium of $50.00 per month. In some cases this amount may be higher if you did not choose Part B when you first became eligible at age 65. The cost of Part B may go up 10% for each 12-month period that you were eligible for Part B but declined coverage, except in special cases. You will have to pay the extra 10% cost for the rest of your life.

Enrolling in Part B is your choice. You can sign up for Part B anytime during a 7-month period that begins 3 months before you turn 65. Visit your local Social Security office, or call the Social Security Administration at 1-800-772-1213 to sign up. If you choose to enroll in Part B, the premium is usually taken out of your monthly Social Security, Railroad Retirement, or Civil Service Retirement payment. If you do not receive any of the above payments, Medicare sends you a bill for your part B premium every 3 months. You should receive your Medicare premium bill in the mail by the 10th of the month. If you do not, call the Social Security Administration at 1-800-772-1213, or your local Social Security office. If you get benefits from the Railroad Retirement Board, call your local RRB office or 1-800-808-0772. For more information, call your Medicare carrier about bills and services. The phone number for the Medicare carrier in your area can be found at the following Web site: **http://www.medicare.gov/Contacts/home.asp**. You may have choices in how you get your healthcare including the Original Medicare Plan, Medicare Managed Care Plans (like HMOs), and Medicare Private Fee-for-Service Plans.

Medicaid

Medicaid is a joint federal and state program that helps pay medical costs for some people with low incomes and limited resources. Medicaid programs vary from state to state. People on Medicaid may also get coverage for nursing home care and outpatient prescription drugs which are not covered by Medicare. You can find more information about Medicaid on the HCFA.gov Web site at **http://www.hcfa.gov/medicaid/medicaid.htm**.

States also have programs that pay some or all of Medicare's premiums and may also pay Medicare deductibles and coinsurance for certain people who have Medicare and a low income. To qualify, you must have:

- Part A (Hospital Insurance),

- Assets, such as bank accounts, stocks, and bonds that are not more than $4,000 for a single person, or $6,000 for a couple, and

- A monthly income that is below certain limits.

For more information, look at the Medicare Savings Programs brochure, **http://www.medicare.gov/Library/PDFNavigation/PDFInterim.asp?Langua ge=English&Type=Pub&PubID=10126**. There are also Prescription Drug Assistance Programs available. Find information on these programs which offer discounts or free medications to individuals in need at **http://www.medicare.gov/Prescription/Home.asp**.

NORD's Medication Assistance Programs

Finally, the National Organization for Rare Disorders, Inc. (NORD) administers medication programs sponsored by humanitarian-minded pharmaceutical and biotechnology companies to help uninsured or under-insured individuals secure life-saving or life-sustaining drugs.[96] NORD programs ensure that certain vital drugs are available "to those individuals whose income is too high to qualify for Medicaid but too low to pay for their prescribed medications." The program has standards for fairness, equity, and unbiased eligibility. It currently covers some 14 programs for nine pharmaceutical companies. NORD also offers early access programs for investigational new drugs (IND) under the approved "Treatment INDs" programs of the Food and Drug Administration (FDA). In these programs, a limited number of individuals can receive investigational drugs that have yet to be approved by the FDA. These programs are generally designed for rare diseases or disorders. For more information, visit **www.rarediseases.org**.

Additional Resources

In addition to the references already listed in this chapter, you may need more information on health insurance, hospitals, or the healthcare system in general. The NIH has set up an excellent guidance Web site that addresses these and other issues. Topics include:[97]

- Health Insurance:
  http://www.nlm.nih.gov/medlineplus/healthinsurance.html

- Health Statistics:
  http://www.nlm.nih.gov/medlineplus/healthstatistics.html

- HMO and Managed Care:
  http://www.nlm.nih.gov/medlineplus/managedcare.html

- Hospice Care: **http://www.nlm.nih.gov/medlineplus/hospicecare.html**

- Medicaid: **http://www.nlm.nih.gov/medlineplus/medicaid.html**

- Medicare: **http://www.nlm.nih.gov/medlineplus/medicare.html**

- Nursing Homes and Long-Term Care:
  http://www.nlm.nih.gov/medlineplus/nursinghomes.html

- Patient's Rights, Confidentiality, Informed Consent, Ombudsman Programs, Privacy and Patient Issues:
  http://www.nlm.nih.gov/medlineplus/patientissues.html

- Veteran's Health, Persian Gulf War, Gulf War Syndrome, Agent Orange:
  http://www.nlm.nih.gov/medlineplus/veteranshealth.html

---

[96] Adapted from NORD: **http://www.rarediseases.org/programs/medication**.
[97] You can access this information at:
http://www.nlm.nih.gov/medlineplus/healthsystem.html.

Vocabulary Builder

The following vocabulary builder provides definitions of words used in this chapter that have not been defined in previous chapters:

Impairment: In the context of health experience, an impairment is any loss or abnormality of psychological, physiological, or anatomical structure or function. [NIH]

Outpatient: A patient who is not an inmate of a hospital but receives diagnosis or treatment in a clinic or dispensary connected with the hospital. [NIH]

ONLINE GLOSSARIES

The Internet provides access to a number of free-to-use medical dictionaries and glossaries. The National Library of Medicine has compiled the following list of online dictionaries:

- ADAM Medical Encyclopedia (A.D.A.M., Inc.), comprehensive medical reference: **http://www.nlm.nih.gov/medlineplus/encyclopedia.html**

- MedicineNet.com Medical Dictionary (MedicineNet, Inc.): **http://www.medterms.com/Script/Main/hp.asp**

- Merriam-Webster Medical Dictionary (Inteli-Health, Inc.): **http://www.intelihealth.com/IH/**

- Multilingual Glossary of Technical and Popular Medical Terms in Eight European Languages (European Commission) - Danish, Dutch, English, French, German, Italian, Portuguese, and Spanish: **http://allserv.rug.ac.be/~rvdstich/eugloss/welcome.html**

- On-line Medical Dictionary (CancerWEB): **http://www.graylab.ac.uk/omd/**

- Technology Glossary (National Library of Medicine) - Health Care Technology: **http://www.nlm.nih.gov/nichsr/ta101/ta10108.htm**

- Terms and Definitions (Office of Rare Diseases): **http://rarediseases.info.nih.gov/ord/glossary_a-e.html**

Beyond these, MEDLINEplus contains a very user-friendly encyclopedia covering every aspect of medicine (licensed from A.D.A.M., Inc.). The ADAM Medical Encyclopedia can be accessed via the following Web site address: **http://www.nlm.nih.gov/medlineplus/encyclopedia.html**. ADAM is also available on commercial Web sites such as Web MD (**http://my.webmd.com/adam/asset/adam_disease_articles/a_to_z/a**) and drkoop.com (**http://www.drkoop.com/**). Topics of interest can be researched by using keywords before continuing elsewhere, as these basic definitions and concepts will be useful in more advanced areas of research. You may choose to print various pages specifically relating to adult acute lymphoblastic leukemia and keep them on file.

Online Dictionary Directories

The following are additional online directories compiled by the National Library of Medicine, including a number of specialized medical dictionaries and glossaries:

- Medical Dictionaries: Medical & Biological (World Health Organization): **http://www.who.int/hlt/virtuallibrary/English/diction.htm#Medical**

- MEL-Michigan Electronic Library List of Online Health and Medical Dictionaries (Michigan Electronic Library): **http://mel.lib.mi.us/health/health-dictionaries.html**

- Patient Education: Glossaries (DMOZ Open Directory Project): **http://dmoz.org/Health/Education/Patient_Education/Glossaries/**

- Web of Online Dictionaries (Bucknell University): **http://www.yourdictionary.com/diction5.html#medicine**

ADULT ACUTE LYMPHOBLASTIC LEUKEMIA GLOSSARY

The following is a complete glossary of terms used in this sourcebook. The definitions are derived from official public sources including the National Institutes of Health [NIH] and the European Union [EU]. After this glossary, we list a number of additional hardbound and electronic glossaries and dictionaries that you may wish to consult.

Ablation: The removal of an organ by surgery. [NIH]

Agarose: A polysaccharide complex, free of nitrogen and prepared from agar-agar which is produced by certain seaweeds (red algae). It dissolves in warm water to form a viscid solution. [NIH]

Antibiotic: A substance usually produced by vegetal micro-organisms capable of inhibiting the growth of or killing bacteria. [NIH]

Apheresis: Components being separated out, as leukapheresis, plasmapheresis, plateletpheresis. [NIH]

Catheters: A small, flexible tube that may be inserted into various parts of the body to inject or remove liquids. [NIH]

CDNA: Synthetic DNA reverse transcribed from a specific RNA through the action of the enzyme reverse transcriptase. DNA synthesized by reverse transcriptase using RNA as a template. [NIH]

Cofactor: A substance, microorganism or environmental factor that activates or enhances the action of another entity such as a disease-causing agent. [NIH]

Compassionate: A process for providing experimental drugs to very sick patients who have no treatment options. [NIH]

Consolidation: The healing process of a bone fracture. [NIH]

Consultation: A deliberation between two or more physicians concerning the diagnosis and the proper method of treatment in a case. [NIH]

Contraindications: Any factor or sign that it is unwise to pursue a certain kind of action or treatment, e. g. giving a general anesthetic to a person with pneumonia. [NIH]

Deletion: A genetic rearrangement through loss of segments of DNA (chromosomes), bringing sequences, which are normally separated, into close proximity. [NIH]

Genetics: The biological science that deals with the phenomena and mechanisms of heredity. [NIH]

Haematology: The science of the blood, its nature, functions, and diseases. [NIH]

Hospice: Institution dedicated to caring for the terminally ill. [NIH]

Immunologic: The ability of the antibody-forming system to recall a previous experience with an antigen and to respond to a second exposure with the prompt production of large amounts of antibody. [NIH]

Impairment: In the context of health experience, an impairment is any loss or abnormality of psychological, physiological, or anatomical structure or function. [NIH]

Infections: The illnesses caused by an organism that usually does not cause disease in a person with a normal immune system. [NIH]

Karyotype: The characteristic chromosome complement of an individual, race, or species as defined by their number, size, shape, etc. [NIH]

Lymphoblastic: One of the most aggressive types of non-Hodgkin lymphoma. [NIH]

Lymphoblasts: Interferon produced predominantly by leucocyte cells. [NIH]

Lymphokine: A soluble protein produced by some types of white blood cell that stimulates other white blood cells to kill foreign invaders. [NIH]

Lymphoma: Tumor of lymphatic tissue. [NIH]

Monoclonal: An antibody produced by culturing a single type of cell. It therefore consists of a single species of immunoglobulin molecules. [NIH]

Morphological: Relating to the configuration or the structure of live organs. [NIH]

MRNA: The RNA molecule that conveys from the DNA the information that is to be translated into the structure of a particular polypeptide molecule. [NIH]

Nerve: A cordlike structure of nervous tissue that connects parts of the nervous system with other tissues of the body and conveys nervous impulses to, or away from, these tissues. [NIH]

Networks: Pertaining to a nerve or to the nerves, a meshlike structure of interlocking fibers or strands. [NIH]

Outpatient: A patient who is not an inmate of a hospital but receives diagnosis or treatment in a clinic or dispensary connected with the hospital. [NIH]

Pharmacodynamic: Is concerned with the response of living tissues to chemical stimuli, that is, the action of drugs on the living organism in the absence of disease. [NIH]

Phenotypes: An organism as observed, i. e. as judged by its visually perceptible characters resulting from the interaction of its genotype with the environment. [NIH]

Polymerase: An enzyme which catalyses the synthesis of DNA using a single DNA strand as a template. The polymerase copies the template in the 5'-3'direction provided that sufficient quantities of free nucleotides, dATP and dTTP are present. [NIH]

Potassium: It is essential to the ability of muscle cells to contract. [NIH]

Probe: An instrument used in exploring cavities, or in the detection and dilatation of strictures, or in demonstrating the potency of channels; an elongated instrument for exploring or sounding body cavities. [NIH]

Protocol: The detailed plan for a clinical trial that states the trial's rationale, purpose, drug or vaccine dosages, length of study, routes of administration, who may participate, and other aspects of trial design. [NIH]

Rankin: A three-bladed clamp. [NIH]

Recombination: The formation of new combinations of genes as a result of segregation in crosses between genetically different parents; also the rearrangement of linked genes due to crossing-over. [NIH]

Reductase: Enzyme converting testosterone to dihydrotestosterone. [NIH]

Refer: To send or direct for treatment, aid, information, de decision. [NIH]

Retrovirus: A member of a group of RNA viruses, the RNA of which is copied during viral replication into DNA by reverse transcriptase. The viral DNA is then able to be integrated into the host chromosomal DNA. [NIH]

Specialist: In medicine, one who concentrates on 1 special branch of medical science. [NIH]

Sperm: The fecundating fluid of the male. [NIH]

Suppression: A conscious exclusion of disapproved desire contrary with repression, in which the process of exclusion is not conscious. [NIH]

Therapeutics: The branch of medicine which is concerned with the treatment of diseases, palliative or curative. [NIH]

Transcriptase: An enzyme which catalyses the synthesis of a complementary mRNA molecule from a DNA template in the presence of a mixture of the four ribonucleotides (ATP, UTP, GTP and CTP). [NIH]

Translocation: The movement of material in solution inside the body of the plant. [NIH]

Triad: Trivalent. [NIH]

Vitro: Descriptive of an event or enzyme reaction under experimental investigation occurring outside a living organism. Parts of an organism or microorganism are used together with artificial substrates and/or conditions. [NIH]

Zoster: A virus infection of the Gasserian ganglion and its nerve branches, characterized by discrete areas of vesiculation of the epithelium of the forehead, the nose, the eyelids, and the cornea together with subepithelial infiltration. [NIH]

General Dictionaries and Glossaries

While the above glossary is essentially complete, the dictionaries listed here cover virtually all aspects of medicine, from basic words and phrases to more advanced terms (sorted alphabetically by title; hyperlinks provide rankings, information and reviews at Amazon.com):

- **The Cancer Dictionary** by Roberta Altman, Michael J., Md Sarg; Paperback - 368 pages, 2nd Revised edition (November 1999), Checkmark Books; ISBN: 0816039542; http://www.amazon.com/exec/obidos/ASIN/0816039542/icongroupinterna

- **Dictionary of Medical Acronymns & Abbreviations** by Stanley Jablonski (Editor), Paperback, 4th edition (2001), Lippincott Williams & Wilkins Publishers, ISBN: 1560534605, http://www.amazon.com/exec/obidos/ASIN/1560534605/icongroupinterna

- **Dictionary of Medical Terms : For the Nonmedical Person (Dictionary of Medical Terms for the Nonmedical Person, Ed 4)** by Mikel A. Rothenberg, M.D, et al, Paperback - 544 pages, 4th edition (2000), Barrons Educational Series, ISBN: 0764112015, http://www.amazon.com/exec/obidos/ASIN/0764112015/icongroupinterna

- **A Dictionary of the History of Medicine** by A. Sebastian, CD-Rom edition (2001), CRC Press-Parthenon Publishers, ISBN: 185070368X, http://www.amazon.com/exec/obidos/ASIN/185070368X/icongroupinterna

- **Dorland's Illustrated Medical Dictionary (Standard Version)** by Dorland, et al, Hardcover - 2088 pages, 29th edition (2000), W B Saunders Co, ISBN: 0721662544, http://www.amazon.com/exec/obidos/ASIN/0721662544/icongroupinterna

- **Dorland's Electronic Medical Dictionary** by Dorland, et al, Software, 29th Book & CD-Rom edition (2000), Harcourt Health Sciences, ISBN: 0721694934, http://www.amazon.com/exec/obidos/ASIN/0721694934/icongroupinter na

- **Dorland's Pocket Medical Dictionary (Dorland's Pocket Medical Dictionary, 26th Ed)** Hardcover - 912 pages, 26th edition (2001), W B Saunders Co, ISBN: 0721682812, http://www.amazon.com/exec/obidos/ASIN/0721682812/icongroupinter na/103-4193558-7304618

- **Melloni's Illustrated Medical Dictionary (Melloni's Illustrated Medical Dictionary, 4th Ed)** by Melloni, Hardcover, 4th edition (2001), CRC Press-Parthenon Publishers, ISBN: 85070094X, http://www.amazon.com/exec/obidos/ASIN/85070094X/icongroupintern a

- **Stedman's Electronic Medical Dictionary Version 5.0 (CD-ROM for Windows and Macintosh, Individual)** by Stedmans, CD-ROM edition (2000), Lippincott Williams & Wilkins Publishers, ISBN: 0781726328, http://www.amazon.com/exec/obidos/ASIN/0781726328/icongroupinter na

- **Stedman's Medical Dictionary** by Thomas Lathrop Stedman, Hardcover - 2098 pages, 27th edition (2000), Lippincott, Williams & Wilkins, ISBN: 068340007X, http://www.amazon.com/exec/obidos/ASIN/068340007X/icongroupinter na

- **Stedman's Oncology Words** by Beverly J. Wolpert (Editor), Stedmans; Paperback - 502 pages, 3rd edition (June 15, 2000), Lippincott, Williams & Wilkins; ISBN: 0781726549; http://www.amazon.com/exec/obidos/ASIN/0781726549/icongroupinter na

- **Tabers Cyclopedic Medical Dictionary (Thumb Index)** by Donald Venes (Editor), et al, Hardcover - 2439 pages, 19th edition (2001), F A Davis Co., ISBN: 0803606540, http://www.amazon.com/exec/obidos/ASIN/0803606540/icongroupinter na

INDEX

JUN 4 2008

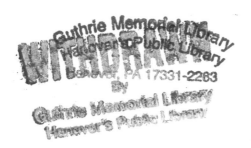
Printed in the United States
110865LV00003B/75/A

9 780497 111847